C000134406

Growing Younger with Yoga

Growing Younger with Yoga

by Louise Wiggins

designed by Simon Anderson-Carr

ISBN: 1 84013 471 2

Copyright © Axiom Publishing, 2001.

This book is copyright. Apart from any fair dealing for the purpose of private study, research, criticism or review, as permitted under the Copyright Act, no part may be reproduced by any process without written permission. Enquiries should be made to the publisher.

This edition for
Grange Books
Units 1-6 Kingsnorth Ind. Est., Hoo, Nr Rochester, Kent ME3 9ND, United Kingdom,
www.grangebooks.co.uk

Publisher's note

Before following any advice or exercises contained in this book, it is recommended that you consult your doctor if you suffer from any health problems or special conditions or are in any doubt as to their suitability. The publisher's, author and the photographer cannot accept responsibility for any injuries or damages incurred as a result of following the exercises in this book.

The images used on pages 8, 12, 13, 14, 17, 52 and 105 were obtained from IMSI's Masterclips Collection, 75 Rowland Way, Novato, CA 94945, USA.

Photograph of Ganesha created by Greg C Grace courtesy of Community Aid Abroad.

The secret of contentment
is knowing how to enjoy what you have.
(Queen Mother aged 99)

People don't grow old,
they become old when they stop growing.
(anon)

My life breath to the immortal wind of spirit.
My body ends in ashes.
(Isa Upanishad)

Contents

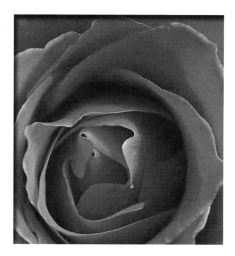

Yoga to Health

Taking the time to smell the roses.
Seeing the rose buds not the thorns.
Letting my life unfold in due season.
Like a bud to bloom in spring.

Remember when? Remember

People are born supple. When they die they are stiff.
Trees are born supple. When they die they are stiff.
Stiffness accompanies death.
Suppleness accompanies life.

(Tao)

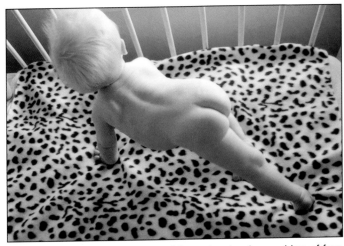

Allow babies and toddlers to remind you of the natural poise and joy of free movement

The next time you have the opportunity to observe a new baby, take a moment to stop and notice the delight with which it explores the space in which it lives. See the joy of free movement, unrestricted by worries, tensions, constriction, contraction, responsibilities and all the other 'straight jacketing' that accompanies so called growing up and growing older.

By all means grow up! But let the timeless wisdom of yoga practices help you grow younger. Make a resolve to remind yourself of your lost flexibility every time a baby comes into your life. You were that flexible once too! It may, however, lie deeply hidden and concealed beneath life's burdens and pressures.

Through a variety of yoga practices, this book will show you how to let the pressures go and rediscover the flexibility that is still there. You'll find the flexibility you gain in yoga is much more than just physical.

Learn to celebrate all movement. Let this new sense of freedom and delight be all the proof you need that there is no need to succumb to the idea that aging relates to deterioration. Be prepared to recondition your beliefs!

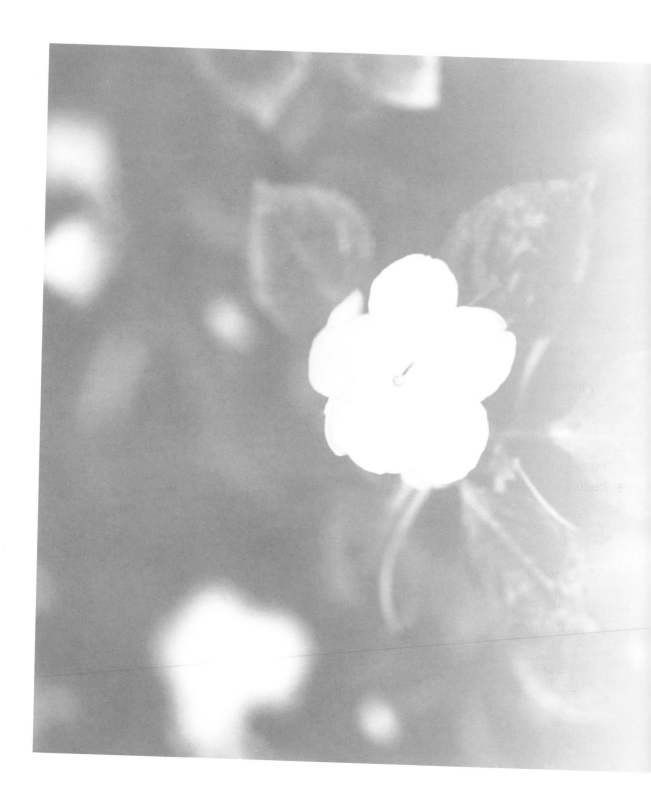

Growing Younger

The King's Command

A romantic legend from the East, tells us how yoga began at the King's court. The King had fallen deeply in love with a beautiful young woman. Her loveliness captivated his heart so much, he became distressed at the thought of her growing older and being ravaged by the hands of time.

The King summoned all the wise men of the land and commanded them to find a way that her beauty and youth could be preserved forever.

After much discussion and thought, the wise men devised the practices of yoga as a system which she could use to hold back the effects of old age.

There is much you can do to feel younger and more energised. This section will not only help you to experience the benefits of yoga practices for the whole body, but also provides proof, life really does begin at 50.

Introduction

Age Not Applicable

When asked her age, Bette simply said, 'not applicable'!

Bette Calman was my first yoga teacher and an inspiration to all her students. I can remember one of the first associations with Bette was at my first yoga class. She had just recovered from a car accident and was sharing with us, some of her experiences. When she was admitted to hospital, and asked to fill in her age, she simply put N/A! As far as Bette was concerned, age was completely irrelevant when it came to healing.

Needless to say her recovery was remarkably rapid. Not only did she not want the doctors to be prejudiced by her age, but she did not want her own preconceived ideas about aging to get in the way of her road to recovery.

I love my age. I allow each day to unfold in peace and stillness.

Our Bodies Were Aging Before We were Ready

I welcome you to the experience of yoga. Like most of my students, I turned to yoga when I was feeling physically unwell and mentally uninspired.

I had just turned 40 and was recovering from some major abdominal surgery. I was overweight, had headaches, suffered arthritic discomfort in many of my joints and was experiencing debilitating sciatica down my left leg. I suddenly felt old! Even my friends were beginning to look old! Geoff, my husband of 15 years, whose lower back was always 'talking' to him, also felt a deterioration in his wellbeing. He was forced to give up playing golf because a simple putt on the green left him immobilised and on the chiropractor's couch. Our bodies were aging before we were ready.

During my convalescent time, I took the opportunity to revisit some of the yoga and meditation books that I had bought years earlier. It was like reading them for the first time. Whereas before, I was focused more on the physical aspects of yoga, I was now able to spend more time on breathing, meditation and relaxation practices. I was able to combine these with my limited physical practices.

I was very grateful for the opportunity to fully realise the healing power of integrated, gentle yoga practices. With improved awareness, I was able to choose gentle yoga stretches to hasten my recovery. To this day I feel eternally grateful for that seemingly negative operation experience. Sometimes we need a setback to hasten our progress. Geoff too, feels a greater power over his own well being. He practices yoga regularly and visits the chiropractor for maintenance reasons rather than therapy.

A Way Of Life

As you introduce yoga into your life, you will find that you begin to make more intelligent, conscious and loving choices that reflect in everything you do. Yoga will become a way of life.

I am so thrilled to be able to guide you through some of the wonderful and timeless yoga practices in this book. Let's enjoy the journey together.

> Yoga teaches
> The body reflects the breath.
> The breath reflects the mind.
> The mind reflects the heart.
> The heart reflects the soul..

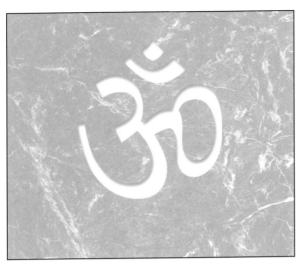

OM is the universal vibration and the sacred symbol of yoga. It represents the three levels of consciousness. The large lower curve represents the dream state, the upper curve the waking state, the curve from the centre, the sleep state. The top curve represents illusion, the dot for transcendence.

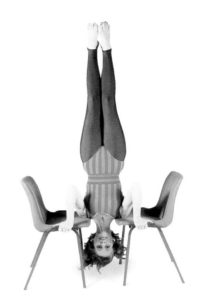

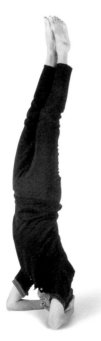

Affirmations

Throughout this book, you will find affirmations to help you on your journey. To get the most benefit from the affirmations, choose one which holds a truth for you and work with that one until it becomes part of your consciousness. Find convenient times during the day to repeat your resolve several times. Perhaps repeating it every time you look at your watch or clock, or every time you make a cup of tea, or every time you stop at a traffic light. Choose something to suit your lifestyle.

I have within me, the power to reach my best potential.

What is Yoga?
Timeless, Ageless

Yoga is an ancient science of wellbeing dating back around 4000 years. It is a time-honoured teaching with its origins in the east. It allow us to experience our best potential at all levels of being. Because it accepts us the way we are, it is suitable to practice at any age and with any level of ability. There are no expectations and no levels of achievement. You won't find it in the Olympics! Yoga is an individual journey of self discovery. It is a unique inner journey which allows you to discover who you really are, exquisitely ageless and timeless. We know this already! You may not have ridden a bicycle for many years. The body you have now, may only vaguely resemble the body which last rode a bike, yet there is a part of you that still knows how to ride a bike. This is the timeless you. This is the real you.

Yoga practices allow us to turn our attention inward so that we can experience ourselves at every level. With improved self awareness, we can make wiser lifestyle choices towards being physically healthy, psychologically strong and mentally at peace.

I am ageless and timeless. I am strong, healthy and at peace.

Wholeness and Healing

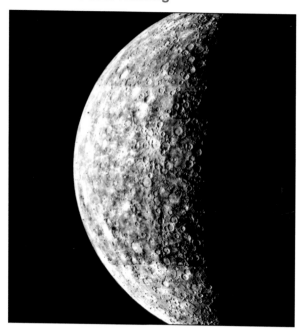

Hatha Yoga is the yoga of postures. 'Ha' means sun. 'Tha' means moon. Hatha yoga is the joining of opposites. The yoking together of all the different aspects of ourselves into a harmonious whole. To heal is to make whole. Yoga heals as it makes us whole. You can discover for yourself the healing power of wholeness as you gently work through your unique body to create a harmoniously functioning whole.

To experience the body as a whole, our yoga practice will include standing and balancing poses, twists, forward and backward bends, side stretches and inversions as well as relaxation, breathing and meditation practices. To get most benefits from your practice, work slowly and gently, with full attention on your free flowing breath and being completely engrossed in the yoga experience. Be fully aware of every moment and every sensation you experience.

You will then have the best opportunity to experience spontaneous healing. Your body will feel revitalised and rejuvenated as the body's processes of digestion, elimination and assimilation are able to work at their optimum levels.

I am aware of the healing power within.

Awareness

Be patient with yourself and have no doubt; yoga really works. Give yourself time to experience yourself as a whole so that you can experience your best potential.

The ultimate aim of yoga is unity and balance; the yoking together of all the different aspects of ourselves into a harmoniously functioning, integrating organism at one with all life. In fact the word yoga is a sanskrit word that means yoke, unite, make one.

Giving yourself your full attention can have amazing results. You may like to try the awareness meditation using almonds on page 94. You'll be surprised how little aware we are most of the time.

I have the patience to allow my best potential to unfold just as it should.

The Classic Yoga Paths

Hatha Yoga
For physical control. It is the yoga of postures and physical well being.

Raja Yoga
The eight fold path as set out by the ancient sage Patanjali. (See P17)

Karma Yoga
The path of selfless service, work and right action, detached from the fruit of the action.

Bhakti Yoga
The path of devotion.

Kundalini Yoga
The path of psychic forces.

Gnana Yoga
The path of wisdom and knowledge.

Mantra Yoga
The path of sound and vibrations. The use of a word, repeated to help focus the mind.

Japa Yoga
The path of repetitive mantras using beads.

Laya Yoga
The path of colours and chakras

Yantra Yoga
The path of mandalas, shapes, symbols and signs

Right Attitude

Yoga teaches that with the right attitude, right action will follow. Do you remember Christopher Reeve, the actor who played in the Superman movies? He had a serious riding accident which left him a quadriplegic and destined for life in a wheelchair. He had the choice of giving up on himself and becoming depressed, or accepting this experience in his life as an opportunity to discover an inner strength and resolve that he didn't know he had. He was determined to realise his best potential, and gave this his full attention. Through effort, intimate awareness and total dedication, he is now very slowly beginning to regain minute sensations in his lifeless body. Whereas we may label these sensations as pain, for Christopher Reeve, they were signs of life and hope.

I focus on being thankful, thankful for all the sensations I experience.

The Power of the Breath

Yoga teaches that breath is life and life is breath. Become intimately acquainted with the power of your breath, letting it enhance and enrich everything you do. When you can harmonise the movements of your body with a free flowing breath, a quiet mind and give it your full attention, you will experience yourself as a whole. And this is yoga.

My mind, my body and my breath are flowing together in the oneness of yoga with all the naturalness with which it was intended.

Choices - Dharmapada

We are what we think.
All that we are arises with our thoughts.
With our thoughts we make the world.
Speak or act with an impure mind
And trouble will follow you
As the wheel follows the ox that draws the cart.

We are what we think.
All that we are arises with our thoughts.
With our thoughts we make the world.
Speak or act with a pure mind
And happiness will follow you
As your shadow unshakable

"Look how he abused me and beat me,
How he threw me down and robbed me."
Live with such thoughts and you live in hate.

"Look how he abused me and beat me,
How he threw me down and robbed me."
Abandon such thoughts, and live in love.

In this world,
Hate never dispelled hate.
Only love dispels hate.
This is the law.
Ancient and inexhaustible.
You too shall pass away.
Knowing this how can you quarrel?

How easily the wind overturns the frail tree.
Seek happiness in the senses,
Indulge in food and sleep,
And you too will be uprooted.

The wind cannot overturn a mountain.
Temptation cannot touch the man
Who is awake, strong and humble,
Who masters himself and minds the law.

If a man's thoughts are muddy,
If he is reckless and full of deceit,
How can he wear the yellow robe?

Whoever is master of his own nature,
Bright, clear and true,
He may indeed wear the yellow robe.

Mistaking the false for the true
And the true for the false,
You overlook the heart
And fill yourself with desire.

See the false as false,
The true as true.
Look into your heart.
Follow your nature.

An unreflecting mind is a poor roof.
Passion like the rain, floods the house.
But if the roof is strong, there is shelter.

Whoever follows impure thoughts
Suffers in this world and the next.
In both worlds he suffers
And how greatly
When he sees the wrong he has done.

Growing Younger

Calming

Whenever you feel flustered, pressured or anxious and you feel the need to calm down, try this simple effective method of creating stillness within.

Choose a word such as calm, peace, serenity, tranquillity, relax, or any other word, suggesting to you the stillness you're looking for.

Sitting quietly with the spine straight and the eyes gently closed, visualise the word written on the screen of your mind at the eyebrow centre between and behind the eyes.

Inhaling through the nostrils, exhale your word allowing it to create ripples of stillness through your whole being, allowing all the cells in your body to absorb the benefits of total relaxation. Immerse yourself in this delicious sensation of stillness and calm.

Yoga teaches

Sanskrit is the ancient language of yoga. It is to the East, what Latin is to the West.

The Astanga Tree of Yoga

The sage **Patanjali** was the first to formulate the practices of yoga into an organised system of 195 brief, condensed statements called 'Sutras'. This system is called 'Astanga Yoga'. Astanga is a sanskrit word literally meaning eight limbs. This system of yoga is therefore often depicted as the limbs of a tree, growing from a solid foundation of wisdom obtained from lifetimes of dedicated meditation on the meaning of life. Patanjali's yoga is also known as Raja (royal) yoga.

Thousands of years ago before books and computers, the precious knowledge of yoga was available only to those who were prepared to spend a lifetime in study. The sacred knowledge was carefully and accurately preserved by a system of passing knowledge from teacher (guru) to student (chela).

4. Pranayama
Breathing practices help us to control prana, which is life force and energy.
I am breathing in, I am breathing out.
I am relaxed.

5. Pratyahara
Practices to help withdraw the senses so that we can experience an inner stillness.
I experience myself in stillness.

3. Asana
The postures of yoga help us to attain a healthy, well functioning, balanced body.
I allow my body to unfold to realise my best potential.

6. Dharana
Concentration practices to help calm the mind.
I am focused. My mind is crystal clear.

2. Niyama
Observances. There are five niyamas which guide us in ethical attitudes and activities towards self discipline. Niyamas are rules for personal conduct.
I am content. I want what I have.

7. Dhyana
Meditation practices to help still the activities of the mind and tune into the natural wisdom of our own true self.
I have trust in the natural intelligence which flows through my body and my mind.

1. Yama
Abstinences. There are five yamas which guide us in moral qualities of word, thought and deed.
I am what I think. I choose my thoughts with care.

8. Samadhi
Self-realisation. A state of union. A realisation that all is one. It is an enlightened state of total bliss and complete knowing.
I am aware. I am awake. I am at peace. I am.

The Eight Limbs Of Yoga
The eight fold path along which the yoga enthusiast embarks on the quest for self-realisation.

The Ten Yoga Guidelines

On the previous page we looked at the eight limbs of yoga. The first two of these limbs are the Yamas and Niyamas. There are five of each and together they give us guidelines for right living.

Yamas - Abstinenses

1. Ahimsa - Non Violence, Harmlessness

Ahimsa means much more than not killing or maiming. It implies compassion and identity with all living creatures, including ourselves. Practicing non-violence means taking care of thought, word and deed, knowing that every act of violence and conflict can be traced back to a single negative thought.

I am what I think. My thoughts serve me well.

2. Satya - Non Lying, Truthfulness

Satya means much more than not telling lies. It reminds us to be truthful about ourselves and others. We will know that truth if we take the time to listen to the intelligence of our inner voice.

I have trust in the silent invisible intelligence which flows through my body and my mind.

3. Asteya - Non Stealing, Honesty

Stealing can take many forms. We can steal someone's self-esteem, accomplishments and joy, just as surely as we can steal his wallet. Not recognising effort and acts of good will and intention, can also be seen as an act of dishonesty.

Today I will give something to everyone I meet. I will give my smile, my appreciation, my gratitude, my time.

4. Bramacharya - Non Lust, Contentment

Being content with what you have, will lead you to wanting what you have and thereby having what you want. Contentment means that we don't waste a lot of our energies on pursuing material possessions.

I am content. I have what I want. I want what I have.

5. Aparigraha - Non Greed, Freedom

Reviewing your attitude towards more and more material possessions, may lead towards an attitude of gratitude that creates a new sense of freedom and space in our life. You will find that you are no longer envious of anyone.

I am grateful for all that I am and all that I have.

Niyamas ...Observances

6. Saucha - Purity

Purity and cleanliness of mind and body includes personal hygiene, healthy eating, and orderly surroundings.

My mind and my body are pure and clean.

7. Santosa - Contentment

As our attitude to life becomes more enlightened, we become more satisfied, strive less and become more healthy.

I am completely satisfied with my mind, my body, my life.

8. Tapas - Self-Discipline

Through self-discipline and burning effort, we will achieve our goals and build strength of character.

I have within me the power and strength to succeed.

9. Svadhyaya - Introspection

Introspection is self-knowledge and self-acceptance, Through a search for wisdom, we will discover the workings of the mind and begin to notice how the ego can be an obstacle to self-fulfilment.

My mind, my body and my breath are flowing together in the oneness of yoga.

10. Ishvara Pranidhana - Humility

Humility is a recognition we are not simply in the natural world, but that we are an integral part of it. It is a yielding to a higher power which flows within us, and through the whole universe.
I surrender.

Yoga teaches

With the right attitude, right thoughts will follow. With the right thoughts, right action. This is karma.

Yoga Stress Busters

1. Join a yoga class
2. Meditate
3. Smile often
4. Make a new friend
5. Rediscover old ones
6. Hug someone
7. Gaze at the stars
8. See beauty everywhere
9. Smell a rose
10. Do some gardening
11. Walk barefoot on the grass
12. Walk in the rain with no umbrella
13. Cuddle your pet
14. Tell those you love, that you do
15. Make a positive resolve
16. Practice relaxation pose
17. Share a problem
18. Try to understand
19. Let someone in
20. Slow your breathing
21. Listen to your breath
22. See new growth
23. Give
24. Give in

Growing Younger - What Can We Do

Henry Ford said, 'Whether you think you can or think you can't, you're right!'
So make a resolve not to limit yourself with thoughts that are negative and counter productive. There is so much we can do if our thoughts are working with us, not against us. The benefits of yoga practices become evident as soon as you begin a regular practice routine. Older students often benefit more because of greater life experience and a higher level of awareness.

1. Acceptance:

Before we can make any constructive changes in our life, we must first of all accept our life the way it is. This releases tension, worries, fears and concerns and allows us to move on. Accept your life and your body as they are now, as a unique expression of all the choices, activities and thoughts of the past. You are the print-out of all this previous programming. Know also that you are the programmer and you have the power to effect any changes in your life that you can conceive of in your mind.

I accept myself just as I am. I rejoice at my growing experience and maturity.

2. Dietary Habits

When we fill our car with fuel, we are always very careful to choose the right petrol or diesel, knowing if we don't, our car's performance will suffer. Isn't it amazing we don't seem to treat our own bodies with this same respect! As you begin to practice yoga regularly, you will slowly begin to honour and respect your own inner intelligence which coordinates and manages such an incredible machine as the human body. You will then begin to make more intelligent and healing choices about what you eat and drink. You'll feel so much better. It is not difficult and your body will love you for it.

I am what I eat. I eat to live, not live to eat.

3. Gentle Yoga Stretches

All yoga stretches are done slowly and gently, allowing you to experience your best potential without limiting yourself or going too far. There is no competition in yoga and no set levels of achievement. It is an intimate exploration of yourself. To get the most benefits from the practices, always allow the breath to be a free flow of energy through your body and your mind. The breath will help you. Experience an energising sensation with each inhalation and a letting go of contraction and tension with each exhalation. Stay with each stretch, breathing deeply and slowly, allowing yourself to explore the very limits of each stretch experience as it applies to your unique body at this time. Listen to your body's natural intelligence to tell you when to move on, stop and rest or stretch further.

I am strong and flexible. I am energetic and enthusiastic.

Yoga teaches

Yoga teaches that peace comes not from doing, but from undoing, not from getting, but from letting go.

4. Stress Management

When you move your mind to your body and allow your breath to be a soft inner focus, something within you shifts towards a greater acceptance of how things are. New ways of handling difficult situations emerge and you find that life is easier, goals more attainable and relationships enriched. Yoga helps you to let go.

I am relaxed and centred. My life is unfolding exactly as it should.

5.Integration

Even just a few minutes invested in some yoga practices will soon pay healthy dividends. Make a resolve to put aside some precious time to be with yourself so that you can experience the integrating effects on your physical and mental wellbeing. You will then experience yourself as a harmoniously functioning whole. It is so easy, because everything you do in your yoga practice is within your own capability. You are never expected to reach a particular level. It is your own unique experience of your body at this time. The movements are done slowly and in harmony with a free flowing breath and a quiet mind.

I am at peace.

6. Putting the Mind back in the Body

Yoga is an inward journey of self-discovery. It is a scientifically designed method of self-exploration, simply by putting the mind back in the body to experience who you really are. Become absorbed in your practice, letting it lure you within. It is a journey of great adventure and we can only do it once! Enjoy the experience of yourself.

I have within me the power to grow and evolve in the direction of my choice.

Growing Younger

Aging

Biologists agree that our biological age potential is about 130! That means when we reach the age of 65, we are really only middle aged!

If we expect to remain active and strong as we age, we will. If we succumb to the belief that we grow frail and weak as we age, we will. Our thoughts and beliefs hold great power over our biology and our growth.

7. Strong Bones

The weight bearing properties of the standing poses will help to build strong bones. The bones need the pull and tug of muscles to become strong, otherwise we invite problems associated with osteoporosis. Men have fewer problems with weakening bones, because their muscles are naturally stronger.

I have the strength to handle anything that comes my way.

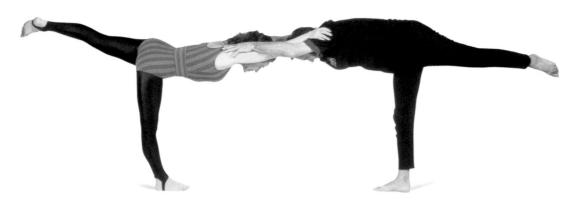

8. Flexibility

Flexibility is achieved when we move all the joints of the body through their maximum range of motion in our pain-free zone. In this way we increase our level of vital energy making us feel absolutely wonderful. As the muscles are lengthened, pockets of tension are released, toxins eliminated as the joints open to receive much needed nourishment. It is a most enjoyable way of keeping the body healthy. We don't want the body to deteriorate just when the mind is beginning to develop. You will find as you become more flexible in your body, you will become more flexible in your attitudes and emotions. Yoga is a fully integrated and holistic practice for the entire being. There is no reason why you shouldn't be more flexible in your seventies than you were in your forties.

I am flexible. I flow with life easily and effortlessly.

9. Your Back

Your spine protects and encloses the whole nervous system connecting your brain to every part of your being, governing and monitoring movement and the wellbeing of the vital organs. No wonder yoga practitioners value the flexibility of the spine so highly.

I am as young as my spine is flexible.

10. Peace of Mind

Combining the breath with relaxation and meditation practices, will help you to be in touch with the stillness which lies within. It is within this stillness that we experience peace of mind.

I am in touch with the stillness within. I am at peace.

11. Breathing

Our breath is the glue which stops us from disintegrating. No wonder yoga practices have breath awareness as a constant inner focus. It is life itself. You will notice an immediate difference if you simply tune into the quality of your breath and allow it to deepen and slow several times a day. Every now and then, stop and notice your breath. See what it tells you. Notice how your breath quickens in times of stress and slows when you are at rest.

I allow my breath to slow, deepen and soften.

12. Meditation

Meditation is inner listening. Take some time each day to sit quietly in a favourite place or a favourite chair, and take some time to listen to your own inner wisdom.

I am calm and relaxed, I have plenty of time for everything.

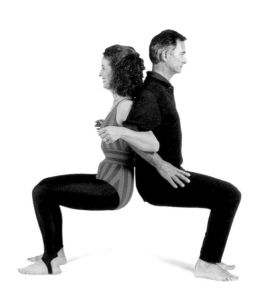

13. Relaxation and Stillness
Learn the technique of body consciousness, by letting your awareness roam around the body so that you can relax those areas touched by your mind. In this way you let go of contractions and tension and experience the inner stillness that is always there.

I surrender to the stillness within.

Ten Commandments for Reducing Stress
1. Thou shalt not be perfect nor even try to be.
2. Thou shalt not try to be all things to all people.
3. Thou shalt leave things undone that ought to be done.
4. Thou shalt not spread thyself too thin.
5. Thou shalt learn to say no.
6. Thou shalt schedule time for thyself and thy supportive network.
7. Thou shalt switch and do nothing regularly.
8. Thou shalt be boring, untidy, inelegant and unattractive at times.
9. Thou shalt not even feel guilty.
10. Especially, thou shalt not be thine own worst enemy, but be thy best friend.

Growing Younger

My breath, my teacher
count your breaths for one minute. If you breathe more than 14-15 breaths per minute, you may be showing signs of stress. Consciously focus on slowing and deepening the breath, releasing the stress.

Garlic Dip
Garlic is a natural and gentle antibiotic and helps to build the body's resistance to disease. It is helpful in eliminating mucus and so will help relieve symptoms of colds. If you love garlic, try this very simple to make garlic dip.

Put in a blender: 1 cup breadcrumbs, 1/2 cup soy milk, 6 cloves of garlic, 3 egg yolks, some parsley and seasoning, 3/4 cup sunflower oil, and the juice of a lemon. Blend until smooth. It will keep in the fridge for about 3 days given half a chance.

Yoga teaches
We are as young as the spine is flexible. Old age begins when we allow the spine to stiffen.

Breathe

Breath is life. Complete breath, complete life. Half breath, half life. No breath, no life. Bliss lies in the effortless suspension of the breath.

Lungs Can't Breathe

The lungs themselves cannot breathe. You need your respiratory muscles to allow the lung tissue to stretch enabling you to breathe in, relax, so that you can breathe out. We have two main sets of breathing muscles. The diaphragm muscle and the intercostal muscles between the ribs. Regular yoga practices will help you develop a way of breathing which is energising, revitalising and yet effortless.

> Yoga teaches
>
> Bliss lies in the effortless suspension of the breath.

The Innocent Breath

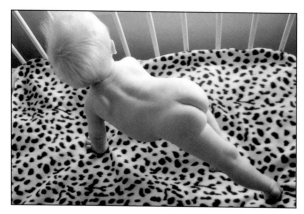

I awoke one night with my little dog fast asleep, stretched lengthwise along the front of my body. His breath was deep, relaxed and innocent. I smiled as I gently rested my hand on his little ribcage and felt privileged to experience his perfectly relaxed breath. He was breathing a beautifully deep, relaxed abdominal breath where the exhalation was a little longer than the inhalation. It helped

me to relax and soon I was back to sleep again. If you have a baby or small child in your life, (or a cuddly little lap dog) take a moment to observe this innocent breath. This is the breath we were all born with. This is the breath we can rediscover when we let go of cares, worries and tensions.

What Is Prana?

Prana is a Sanskrit word meaning vital energy, or life force. When we breathe in, we breathe in prana and air. When we breathe out we breathe out only air. So you can see the importance of breathing practices in yoga.

> Yoga teaches
>
> Yoga teaches that prana is the essential life force which glues the cells together. Without the presence of prana the body decomposes and dies.

The Energising Breath

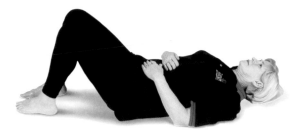

Lie down in the semi supine position with the knees bent and both the knees and feet in line with the hips. Place your left hand below the navel, on the pelvic triangle. Place

The Benefits of Yogic Breathing With Awareness

- Tension is released and the body relaxes.
- Vitality is increased, overcoming fatigue.
- Efficient oxygen supply purifies the blood.
- Memory and concentration is improved.
- Sleeping and mental processes are facilitated.
- Improved metabolism will help control body weight.
- Vitality will show in bright eyes and skin tone.
- Healthier lung tissue will resist disease.
- You won't catch as many colds.
- Waste products are more efficiently eliminated.
- Your whole body will be better nourished.
- Deep breathing gives you an inner massage.
- Diaphragm movement stimulates the liver and inner organs as it gently massages the heart.
- Posture is improved as the chest opens and shoulders broaden.
- You'll feel uplifted and more energetic.
- Deep rhythmic breathing provides a calm inner focus for the preparation of meditation.
- The nerves relax as anxiety is replaced by an inner peace and calm.
- It feels so good!

the right hand on the sternum with the last 2 fingers resting on the solar plexus. Monitor your breath, observing the movement you feel beneath both hands. Plenty of movement under the right hand, very little under the hand resting on your well toned lower abdomen. Take a moment to experience the connection between the breath and the diaphragm.

Breath Awareness in Crocodile Pose *Makarasana*
Rest in the prone position with the forehead resting on the back of the hands, fingers overlapping, elbows wide and in line with each other. Use this pose to enrich your experience of your deep, natural breath flow.

Feel it in the solar plexus, and let it relieve tension in the back. Notice how your breath has naturally deepened. Feel the solar plexus press into the floor with each in breath and retract with each out breath.

My body, my mind, and my breath flow together in perfect harmony.

Understanding the Energising Breath

Study the two diagrams below. It will help you understand how to breathe energetically with a gently toned abdomen. Begin your awareness with an exhalation. At the end of your exhalation, gently but firmly draw in the lower abdomen (below the navel), then holding on to the gentle strength in the lower abdomen, breathe into the solar plexus (the belly above the navel) and rib cage. When you're ready, breathe out solar plexus, rib cage. Observe the function of the diaphragm and abdomen in breathing. Give it your full attention.

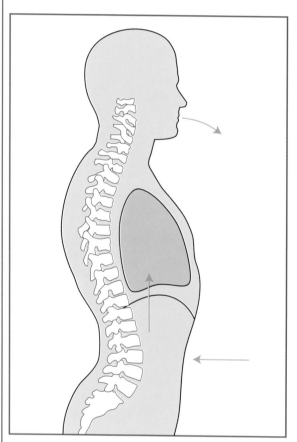

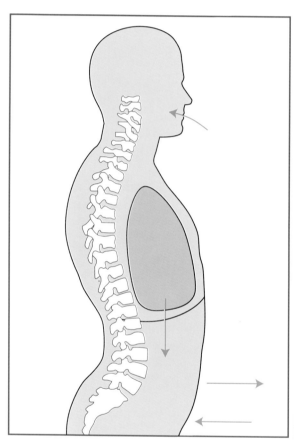

Exhalation

As you exhale, allow the breath to flow from the solar plexus, while still keeping the lower abdomen gently toned. Notice how the breath tends to be more complete, allowing more stale air and toxins to be squeezed out as the diaphragm is assisted by your firmly toned abdominal wall.

Inhalation

As you inhale, allow the breath to flow into the solar plexus, while keeping the lower abdomen gently toned. In this way the viscera are supported, while breathing deeply. The digestive organs will also be gently massaged into activity. Feel energy and vitality flow in on the breath. Experience it in your own unique way.

Pranayama

Prana is life force – ayama is to control. Pranayama practices help us to control the flow of life force through the body. Try these three pranayama practices and experience for yourself, new levels of energy and vitality.

1. The Ujjayi Breath

Begin in the semi-supine position with the low back resting, shoulders broad and away from the ears and the back of the neck long and relaxed. You may need a small cushion to be more comfortable.

Focus on your natural relaxed breath. Focus on the back of the throat and imagine you are trying to whisper 'ahh' behind your closed lips. Experience the contraction in the back of the throat. Continue to breathe with this contraction gently held on both the inhalation and the exhalation. Notice the gentle purring sound with each breath. Let the sound of your own breath give you a soft inner focus as you allow the breath to deepen and lengthen.

When you're ready, experience the spaces between the breath and the stillness there. This is a perfectly natural suspension of your breath. Linger for a moment in the stillness of the pause. Allow the pause to lengthen of its own accord, without any strain or tension, but simply giving it your full attention. Explore how deep and full you can make your breath. Use the ujjayi breath in any of your postures.

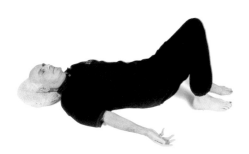

2. Nadi Sodhana The Alternate Nostril Breath

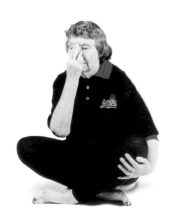

Sitting upright on the floor or on a chair. Elongate the space between the pubis and the sternum lengthening and straightening the spine.

When you're ready, place your right thumb near the right nostril, the next two fingers between the eyebrows and the last two fingers near the left nostril with the head in a natural reading position, shoulders relaxed.

Close the right nostril with the thumb, inhale through the left nostril, lightly close the left nostril, exhale right. Inhale right, close right nostril with the thumb and exhale left. This is one round. Continue this practice for a few minutes, enjoying the benefits of uniting all the opposing aspects of yourself and immersing yourself in the experience of your breath. The alternate nostril breath creates mental clarity, and inner balance and harmony as it purifies the nadis (subtle energy channels in the body).

3. The Complete Breath

Beginning in the semi-supine position as before, rest both hands on the solar plexus, between the navel and the sternum. Take a moment to allow the breath to deepen and relax you more with each exhalation. Visualise the lungs as pear-shaped vessels that will fill from the wide bottom to the narrower top, divided roughly into three portions.

Experience the breath deepen into the base of the lungs only. Feel it lift the abdomen beneath your hands. Enjoy the experience of this deep relaxed diaphragmatic breath. Your innocent breath.

When you're ready, move your hands on the sides of the rib cage and experience the movement. Rest your hands on the collar bones and as the breath deepens even more, experience the shoulder girdle expanding up towards the ceiling.

With the exhalation, breathe out lower, middle then upper portions of the lungs. Continue to experience at least five more rounds of the complete breath. Enjoy the experience of being fully alive!

The belly moves out as you breathe in and moves in as you breath out.

The Benefits of Correct Breathing

- Relaxing and releasing tension
- Energising and overcoming fatigue
- Increasing energy levels and vitality
- Improving sleep patterns
- Improving circulation to the brain helping memory
- Sharpening mental activity
- Improving metabolism, thereby controlling weight
- Clearing skin
- Resisting disease
- Massaging the inner organs
- Feeling uplifted
- Brightening the eyes
- Lifting the mood
- Calming the mind
- Slowing the breath, increasing life expectancy
- Calming the nervous system
- Allowing angry words to remain unspoken
- Replacing fear with love
- Being centred in stillness

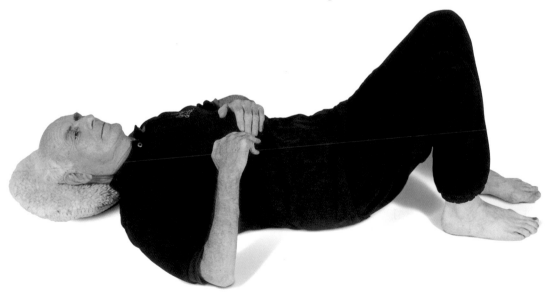

Moving Breath Meditation

This simple two breath meditation practice will give you a profound sensation of peace and well being. Wherever possible enjoy this practice outdoors, in the garden or in a place of natural beauty.

Preparation
Mountain Pose (see P52) with the knees soft, shoulders relaxed, face, eyes, throat at ease and the back of the neck lengthening, chin slightly drawn in.

1. Inhale
I gather it all up.
Allowing the arms to widen and reach upwards to explore the space around you. Reach for your best potential, your dreams, your aspirations; gathering it all up.

2. Exhale
I direct it to the centre of my being.
Direct it slowly down through the centre of your body and let it settle and rest in the hara centre just below and behind the navel.

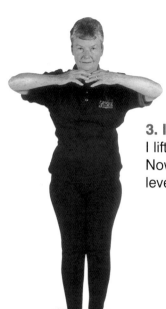

3. Inhaling

I lift it to my heart.

Now turning the palms up and slowly and gently lifting it up to the level of the heart, allowing it to permeate the heart centre.

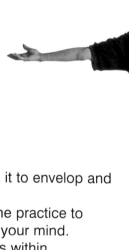

4. Exhaling

I spread it all around.

Then spreading it all around you, allowing it to envelop and enfold you.

   Repeat 1-4 several times more. Allow the practice to naturally deepen your breath and quieten your mind. Experience a deep inner calm and stillness within.

Yoga teaches

Yoga teaches that where the mind goes, energy flows. Allow the mind to direct the energy wherever it is most needed. Allow your body to respond.

Growing Younger

Stillness

During meditation, breathing and relaxation practices, you will be able to experience the benefits of stillness within the body and the mind. Stillness fills the spaces between the cells as water surrounds the pebbles at the bottom of the pond. Allow the stillness to permeate the cells of the body and the mind, absorbing tension, negativity, and unwanted thought patterns. Letting it all go. Letting it float away in the vast spaciousness of your awareness.

The Anti-Anxiety Breath

Growing younger by curing the 'hurry-hurry' disease.
Here is the perfect antidote to the 'hurry-hurry' epidemic! Banish this infliction by breathing in harmony with your own natural inner wisdom. Here's how.

The 'Hurry-Hurry' Disease

Have you caught the hurry bug? Always rushing and never making time for yourself? This disease is very infectious, and very prevalent in our society today! The breath provides us with the medicine and cure by allowing us to tune into the natural healing force within.

I am aware that treatment comes from the outside, healing comes from within.

Stillness

Stillness lies beneath all the activities, all the busy-ness of our daily lives. It is always there, waiting patiently for us to come and visit. All we have to do, is be aware of its existence and take the time to stop and turn our awareness within.

In stillness I heal.

The Anti-Anxiety Breath

Find a comfortable place to sit or lie down, where you won't be disturbed.

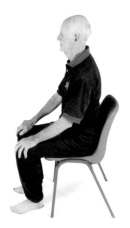

Allow the spine to be straight and aligned, head directly in line with the shoulders. Close the eyes. Let go. When you're ready, tune into the natural ebbing and flowing of your relaxed breath. Accept the breath just as it is at this time. Be aware of any sensations you experience. Very gently, let your breath deepen into the belly of its own accord. Experience the solar plexus, rising and falling. Make no effort to control the breath. Simply let the breath emerge and grow in its own time. Inhalation, belly rising, exhalation, belly falling. Notice how the breath wants to deepen even more. You'll now experience it as an expansion in the rib cage. Let it deepen. Let it grow. Let go your need to control for a few moments. Inhaling belly, ribcage. Exhaling belly, ribcage.

When your breath is ready to deepen more, allow it to more into the upper reaches of the lungs. No tension, no effort. Simply letting the breath grow and mature in its own good time.

Tune into the breath's natural intelligence, telling you exactly the right time to finish the inhalation, pausing just a moment before inviting you to breathe out. Linger within the pauses between the breaths, letting them lengthen if they want to. Linger in the exquisite experience of being in perfect harmony with your body's natural intelligence. It knows just what's right for you at this time.

> ### Yoga teaches
> Yoga teaches that at birth we are given a certain number of breaths. So lengthening your breath will lengthen your life.

Allow yourself to experience the full healing benefits of this deep calm breath. Linger in the stillness of the pause, knowing that bliss lies within the effortless suspension of the breath.

Lion Pose *Simsanasa*

Guard your stillness and roar away aggression in Lion Pose. Sitting back on the heels, arms and fingers fully stretched. Open your bulging eyes wide, inhale then stick out your tongue, exhale and roar loudly! Experience a wonderful deep release within a determined inner strength. Repeat as often as necessary!

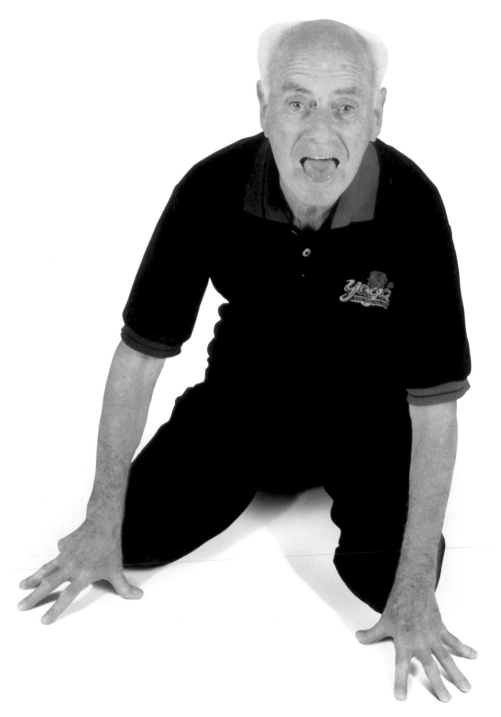

Loving the Heart

Your heart needs both exercise and rest. It loves to work and it loves to rest. Exercise it using conscious yoga postures without strain and without holding the breath. Rest it by inverting the body so that the venous blood can return effortlessly back to the heart.

The Mouse and the Elephant
Our respiratory rate is directly related to the heart rate. Slow respiratory rate slows the heart rate. A slow heart beat is conducive to long life. Just look at the long living elephants with a heart beat of 25 beats per minute compared to the short life span of a mouse with a heart rate of 1000 beats per minute.

Two Snuggling Pumps
The heart is really two muscular pumps snuggled side by side to the left of centre of the chest. The left pump receives blood from the lungs and pumps it into the arteries. The veins return the blood to the right side of the heart. It is interesting that by the time the blood has reached the veins, the blood pressure has dropped to almost zero. The veins are left to direct the blood back to the heart. It does this by the combined effort of the valves inside the veins, the skeletal muscles, especially in the legs, and the diaphragm muscle as we breathe.

Breathe, Relax, Invert
So you can see how yoga can benefit the heart by breathing practices, relaxation techniques and inversions. Practice the Anti-Anxiety breath on p31 and the Ujjayi breath on p27 to help you slow down the breathing.

Your Heart Knows How To Relax
Each heart beat consists of .3sec work and .5sec rest. In this way it can keep going for a lifetime. So you can see that rest is natural. Learn from the wisdom of your heart.

2500 Million Beats
During a lifetime of 70 years, the heart beats in excess of 2500 million beats, pumping the blood through about 100,000km of blood vessels. It is such a hard working, precious organ.

Loving the Heart
The heart is an active muscle needing its own blood supply which it gets through the coronary arteries. So keep the blood healthy by reducing fat intake and drinking more water. Eat less refined foods, don't add salt, smoke or be overweight. Take time to relax and learn how to breathe.

Yoga For Your Heart

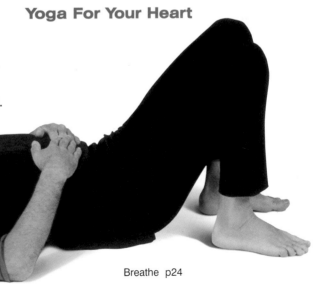

Breathe p24

33

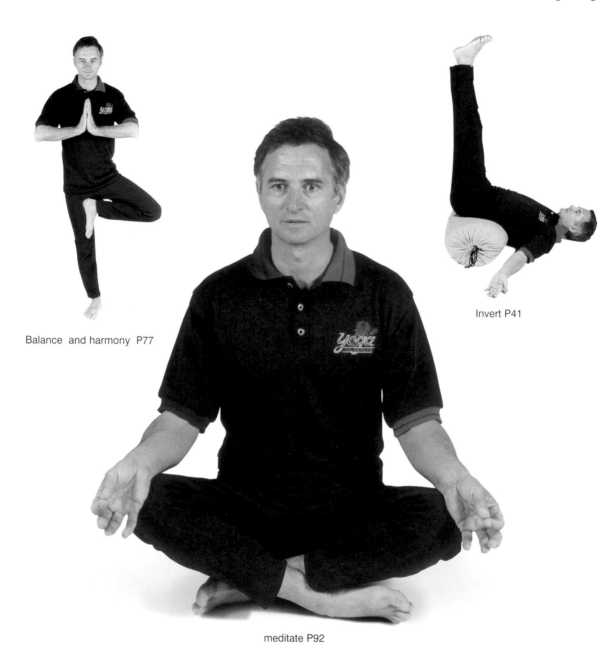

Balance and harmony P77

Invert P41

meditate P92

Growing Younger

Living Longer

The ancient yogis spent much time in nature, observing animals in great detail. You'll notice many of the yoga poses are named after animals. The yogis noticed that the slow breathing animals such as snakes, elephants and tortoises lived longer than the rapid breathing rabbits, mice and birds.

A slower beating heart lives longer. Knowing that the rate at which we breathe is directly related to the pulse, make a resolve to slow your breathing to benefit the heart.

Asthma and Breathing Problems

- Yoga practices improve the wellbeing of the whole body, improving resistance to disease.
- You will find your breathing techniques are greatly enhanced.
- You won't believe the incredible improvement you'll experience simply by breath awareness practices.

Yoga practices improve our breathing techniques and this will benefit the well being of the whole body.

Through regular yoga practices using your breath intelligently, you will increase your level of awareness to help you identify those trigger factors affecting you. Breathing problems can be reversed through improved mobility of the chest muscles, abdominal strength, relaxation techniques, stress relief, breathing and improved posture. Yoga helps to create inner harmony and wholeness. This wholeness is health and ease. Disharmony causes illness which is dis-ease.

Asthma

Asthma creates breathing difficulties because the air passages (the bronchi) may contract as they are under nervous control. The airways narrow during an attack. Infections, allergies and stress are amongst the main triggers. When the muscular walls of the air passages spasm, there will be a feeling of tightness in the chest and a shortage of breath. This leads to anxiety and wheezing as the body looks for more air. When this happens, it is common to hold onto the inhalation, grasping the air and holding it in. Asthmatics commonly have difficulty breathing out and letting go. This is where yoga breathing and relaxation techniques are so helpful. You can see from the following diagrams how air passages are reduced when the airways muscles spasm.

Your Breath

Also see the 'Anti-Anxiety Breath' on P31 and the Soft Blowing Breath' on P37. Tune into your natural breath. Stress and tension are important triggers. Once you've tuned into your natural complete breath, observing it in stillness, allow the exhalation to gently lengthen, making sure the face and shoulders are relaxed. Learn to relax the breathing muscles. Simply take a few moments at any time of the day to tune into the quality of your breath. Just by watching it, you'll find it will soften, deepen and relax of its own accord. The body wants to heal itself, it wants to be well.

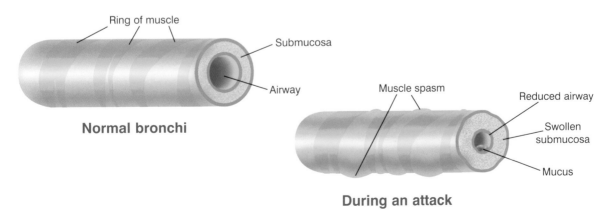

Ring of muscle
Submucosa
Airway

Normal bronchi

Muscle spasm
Reduced airway
Swollen submucosa
Mucus

During an attack

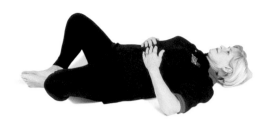

Tuning into your natural relaxed breath, lying down to relax the diaphragm.

Growing Younger

Healthy Hints

• Improve your posture. Poor posture promotes poor breathing.

• Eat plenty of fresh food and vegetables

• Drink eight glasses of water a day to reduce the viscosity of the mucus.

• Pineapple fruit or juice, is an excellent natural antiseptic.

• Learn how to meditate

The Relaxation Breath

Sitting upright with the spine straight and supported. As you inhale slowly through the nostrils, mentally say to yourself, 'I am breathing in'. When you're ready to exhale slowly through the nostrils, mentally say to yourself, 'I am breathing out'.

Gently experience the pause at the end of the exhalation. Linger in the pause for a moment as you mentally say to yourself, 'I am relaxed'. Repeat five times more.

Postures To Open the Chest
• See p110 for a simple daily practice routine.
• Relaxation pose, to let go tension and relax the shoulders and chest. See p96
• Side stretch to open the side ribs see p87
• The 7-Way Stretch to loosen the whole spine p120
• Sphinx pose for a gentle back bend see p79
• Mountain pose for better posture see p52
• Child pose for a gentle forward bend see p80
• Inversion to help drain the mucus. See Ironing Board Slope and Play Ball on p58-59
• Meditation for stillness and calm and listening to the natural wisdom within. p92
• Have Fun and improve your circulation with the rebounder p123

Chest Opener and Expander
Roll a large towel or a thin blanket into a tight roll, long enough to support your torso and head. You may need a small cushion under the head. In the picture, Joyce is using a bolster. Breathe and allow the chest to expand. Experience the chest opening and expanding with each exhalation.

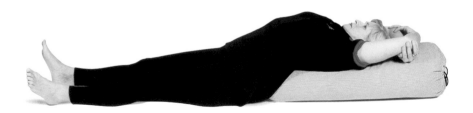

Chest expander, with optional arms overhead

The Soft Blowing Breath

Have you noticed that when you feel anxious, the breath is very rapid and shallow and you're hardly breathing out at all? Practice this Soft Blowing Breath at any time so that you can blow away any anxiety. Your body will feel nourished as you pay attention to its needs.

Turning your attention to the breath, experience the inhalation as a cool gentle stream of nourishment through the nostrils up into the nasal cavities and then within. When you're ready to exhale, make a small (kiss like) hole with the lips and breath out a soft, round, long relaxation breath, letting go all the tension and negativity that you need not hang on to any longer.

Growing Younger
Laugh anyway!

Laughter really is the best medicine. Laughter floods the system with endorphins, the feel good hormones. So even if you don't feel happy, laugh anyway! Your body won't know the difference! Laughter is also the antidote to stress. Laughter stimulates the parasympathetic ('p' for peace) nervous system, creating a natural balance for the sympathetic ('s' for stress) nervous system.

So enjoy happy times with friends and have a good belly laugh every day! As an added bonus, you'll notice that you won't feel pain while you're laughing.

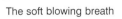

The soft blowing breath

As I breath in, I breath in healing and calming energies,
As I breath out, I let go of tension, tightness and negativity.

Bones and Joints

- After the Skylab astronauts spent 211 day in space in 1973, they came back with osteoporosis and weakened bone tissue. Bone tissue is alive and needs weight bearing to be strong.
- Bones are strengthened when muscles pull and tug on your skeleton.
- So move it or lose it.
- Continuous passive motion as experienced in gentle yoga stretches will actually regenerate cartilage for healthy joints.

Arthritis

Arthritis is soreness and inflammation in the joints of the body. Osteoarthritis develops when the cartilage in a joint wears away. When the cartilage wears away, the surfaces of the bones rub together without the protection of the smooth cartilage. In rheumatoid arthritis the cartilage is also worn away but in this case is replaced by scar tissue which may result in a joint fusing, causing stiffness and pain.

Move It Or Lose It

Arthritis needs exercise, moving the joints through their best range of motion. Find something you enjoy. Walk, swim, dance and yoga to health. Arthritis often develops as a result of poor diet, stress, lack of exercise and lack of sunshine. Lack of exercise causes more stiffness and more imbalance in the body. So keep the joints moving within your pain free zone to keep the joints mobile and nourished.

Also see Practice Routine 1 on p110 Moving it, not losing it in dog pose to strengthen bones and avoid rounded shoulders (kyphosis)

Growing Younger

Worrying

We spend about 99% of the time worrying about things that will probably only happen about 1% of the time.

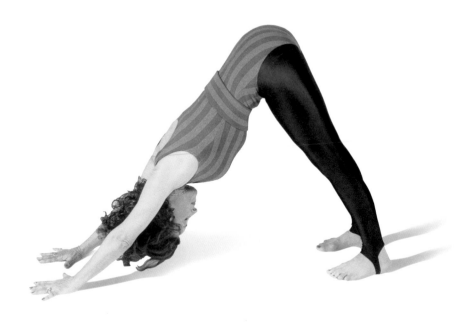

Osteoporosis

Without weight bearing exercise, your bones will become porous just like those of the astronauts. As bone density is lost, breakdown of bone tissue exceed repair, risking osteoporosis. The bones become porous and brittle and fractures occur more easily. Because bone tissue is alive, we can do much to help. The best prevention is to ensure the diet has enough calcium, magnesium, phosphorus and vitamins A, C and D to help absorption. You may like to visit your natural health practitioner for possible dietary supplements.

Move It Or Lose It

When we move, we use muscles, which strengthen with use. Strong muscles pull strongly on the bones to help build bone tissue. So move your body to develop strength and flexibility for strong bones and healthy joints.

You will greatly benefit from some very simple lifestyle changes. Practice the 'Strength' poses on p64 and the Practice Routine 3 on p116. Have fun with the 'rebounder' p123. Make sure to include calcium rich foods in your diet. Foods such as dark green vegetables, almonds, sesame seeds and tahini, low fat dairy products and calcium fortified foods.

Avoid Acid Forming Food

Acid forming foods dissolve calcium from the bones and may deposit it in the joints to form spurs. So cut down or avoid, salt, sugar, red meat, caffeine.

Everything in my life is in perfect order. My life is unfolding just as it should.

Vitamin D regulates the absorption of calcium, so greet the sun everyday.

Blood Pressure

High blood pressure is known as hypertension. Reduced salt intake, a return to normal weight, gentle yoga stretches, and relaxation practices can usually help to return blood pressure to normal. Work in consultation with your health practitioner especially if you feel you may be able to reduce medication. Yoga practices will help you balance all the body functions and bring back a state of equilibrium.

Stress

During situations you consider stressful, adrenaline is released. This in turn increases heart rate and blood pressure.

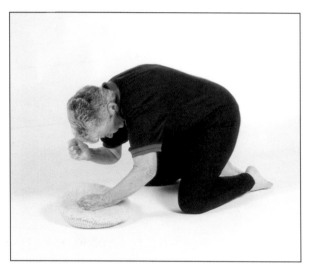

Pummel Your Pillow

As well as diet, stress can increase blood viscosity, increasing blood pressure. So find ways to release tension. If you don't want to take up boxing, pummel your pillow, beat the ground, stamp your feet, scream into the wilderness, letting it go, taking it out of your body without taking out on your loved ones. You may also like to try the Lion Pose on p32.

Only One Cell Thick

The wall thickness of the finest capillary is only a single cell thick. In fact, it can only be seen under a light microscope. The total length of the blood vessels in our body is many thousands of kilometres. So keeping the blood thin and pure will benefit the whole circulatory system; the system that endlessly and faithfully delivers nutrients and removes toxins from the body.

Enjoy The Following Yoga Postures Without Strain, Breathing Easy.

Breathe, meditate and balance poses as in 'Loving the Heart'. Remember to never strain or hold your breath. Be careful not to lower the head below the level of the heart.

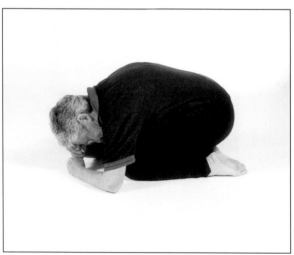

Child pose (P55) with forehead raised, surrender, let go.

Growing Younger

Eavesdropping

Your body is constantly eavesdropping on your mind.

Research has shown that if you suffer from frequent attacks of happiness and laughter, are satisfied with your job and take care of cholesterol levels, you're are much less likely to encounter heart disease.

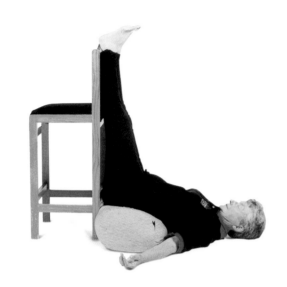

Invert, with legs up the wall. Experiment with elevating the buttocks a little by sitting on the back of your hands or using a bolster as shown by Colleen.

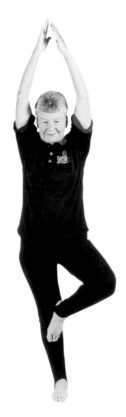

Helpful Hints

- Drink lots of fresh filtered water.
- Eat less fats and refined foods. 'Fat' blood is thick blood.
- Take time to relax.
- Visualise your blood vessels opening and relaxing a little more with each exhalation.
- Start a new hobby or learn a new skill.
- Avoid postures that cause strain. Breathe easily and rhythmically.
- Cut down on refined carbohydrates such as sweets, white flour and sugar. It will help thin the blood.
- Cut down on smoking, alcohol, caffeine.
- Meditate regularly
- Avoid inversions where the head is below the heart.

Yoga Stress Busters

1. Give someone something
2. Give a smile
3. Give a compliment
4. Give affection
5. Give your attention
6. Give your gratitude
7. Make time for yourself
8. Stretch your body
9. Keep a promise
10. Don't give up

Seven Times Seven...Life Begins At 50!

Yoga teaches that there are 7 main centres in the body for the collection of life force. These centres are called chakras. There are 7 notes in the musical scales, there are 7 colours in the rainbow.

   If we allow each chakra to represent 7 years, we can see how life really does begin at 50!

The 7 Chakras

The chakras are energy centres in the body for the collection of life force. Maximum energy will be available to us when the body is in balance and in harmony. Regular yoga practices will help us to maximise the energy available to us at any time. You will experience an inner radiance which is noticeable to others.

   Yoga also teaches that we have 7 such energy centres in the body located in alignment with the spinal column. It is interesting that they correspond with the ductless glands that make up the endocrine system. The accompanying diagram shows the relationship between the chakras and the endocrine system.

   For optimum health and vitality, we need a free flow of energy along this vital axis of the body.

   As we mature, we open ourselves to greater levels of awareness. Our needs move from basic, earthbound energies, to physical and emotional maturity, to greater insight and higher levels of consciousness.

Growing Up

This growing awareness corresponds surprisingly well to 7 year spans at each chakra level. As we age we literally grow up! Once each level of maturation has been experienced, we can enjoy our new found wisdom and focus our later years on fine tuning our organism into the vehicle that best serves our own unique purpose in life.

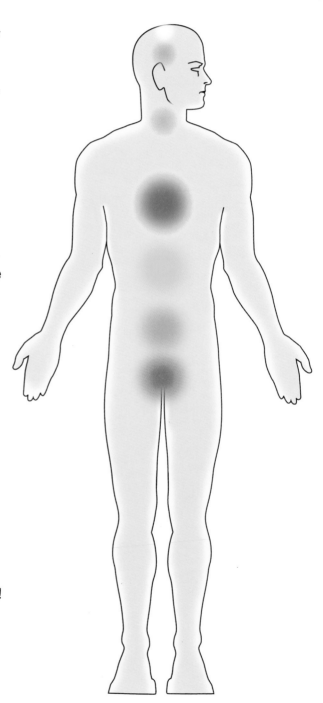

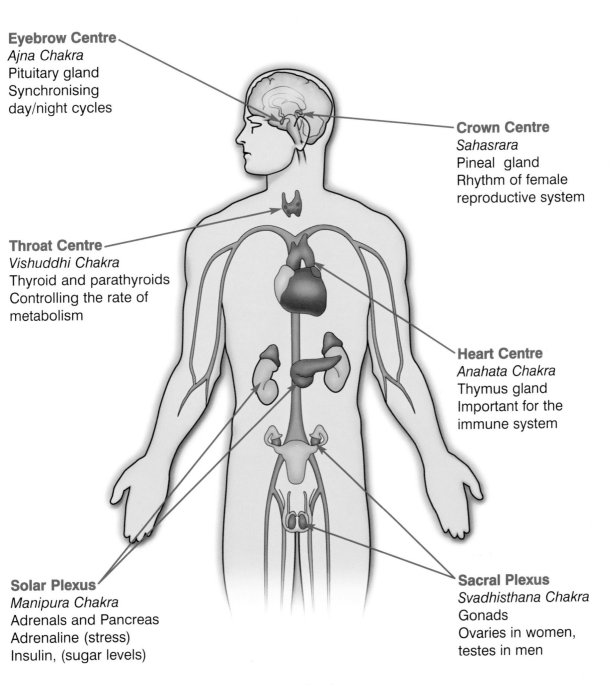

Eyebrow Centre
Ajna Chakra
Pituitary gland
Synchronising
day/night cycles

Crown Centre
Sahasrara
Pineal gland
Rhythm of female
reproductive system

Throat Centre
Vishuddhi Chakra
Thyroid and parathyroids
Controlling the rate of
metabolism

Heart Centre
Anahata Chakra
Thymus gland
Important for the
immune system

Solar Plexus
Manipura Chakra
Adrenals and Pancreas
Adrenaline (stress)
Insulin, (sugar levels)

Sacral Plexus
Svadhisthana Chakra
Gonads
Ovaries in women,
testes in men

Base Chakra
Muladhara Chakra
Not an obvious link to the
endocrine system

Seven Sevens

First 7 years...base chakra
In these young years we are mainly concerned with our basic needs of shelter, safety, food, security. We develop a strong connection to the earth moving from crawling to upright posture, eager to begin the exploration of our environment.

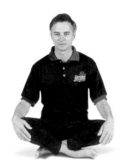

Simple Sitting Pose
I am grounded, safe, secure. I am alive. I love the life I lead

Second 7 years....sacral plexus
From the age of 7 to the adolescent years, we experience an awakening of our identity as a creative being. Here we experience the awakening of our sexuality as we reach puberty.

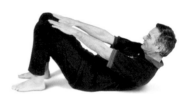

Abdominal Strength
I am creative and productive. I am growing. I am me.

Third 7 years... solar plexus
As we move towards our early twenties, we experience an awakening of our emotional needs. We develop an inner sense of personal power and knowing. These are our gut feelings.

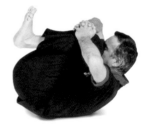

Spine Stretch
I trust my inner knowing. I am in tune with my inner feelings.

Fourth 7 years...heart centre
When in our twenties, we generally feel the need to integrate the first 3 energy levels of security, physical and emotional maturity and settle down, fall in love, marry and have children.

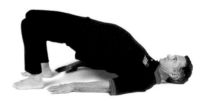

Bridge Pose
I love my family, my friends, my life, myself.

Fifth seven years...throat centre
In our early to mid thirties we develop the need to speak up for ourselves. We experience a growing need to express our unique selves. It is our centre of communication.

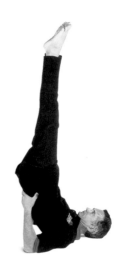

Half Shoulder Stand
I speak my mind. I speak with love from the heart.

Sixth 7 years...Eyebrow centre
In our early forties, we are more likely to experience a growing awareness of our emotional and psychological maturity as we develop awareness and trust in our own inner guru, our own natural intelligence, intuitive wisdom and insight.

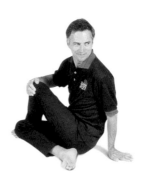

Spinal Twist
I see clearly. I see my purpose. I see my life unfolding just as it should.

Seventh 7 years
As we approach fifty, we develop a growing awareness of our higher self, knowing that we are much more than just our body. We begin to awaken to the experience of who we really are; ageless, timeless and ever lasting, at one with the universe.

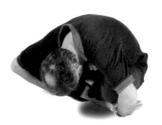

Yoga Mudra
I am. I am at peace. I am content. I am.

Grow old along with me! The best is yet to be. The last of life for which the first was made. (Robert Browning)

Geoff Wiggins 56

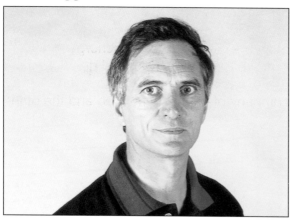

Geoff began regular yoga classes 6 years ago. He has found it of great benefit for the strength of his low back. It has given him self management tools and greater awareness of situations that may cause the onset of a back-attack. As an accountant and author, Geoff spends many hours at the computer terminal and values the postural benefits of yoga practices. It has given him a new sense of power over his own well being.

Joyce Quin 63

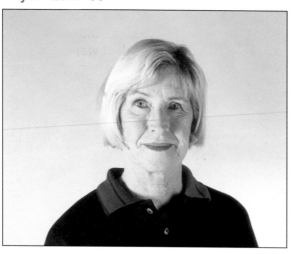

Joyce has been practicing yoga for 7 years and finds herself more flexible and energetic now than ever before. Joyce finds she has greater energy for her family and interests. The breathing, relaxation and awareness practices helped Joyce to make a speedy recovery after some recent foot surgery. When Joyce sold her Real Estate business, yoga provided her with much needed relaxation skills and new levels of fitness and well being.

Colleen Booker 72

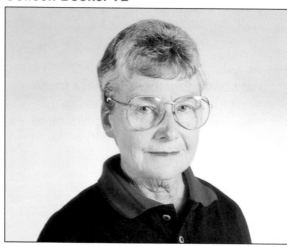

Colleen began practicing yoga regularly when she was in her late 50s. Her lovely upright posture reflects one much younger. She started yoga because of back problems. After years of physiotherapy to release pinched nerves, Colleen now has the tools for self health management. In fact she has not needed to visit the physiotherapist for almost a year now. Colleen enjoys excellent health allowing her to continue do the things she loves such as swim and travel extensively with her husband Tony. She attends regular yoga classes with her daughter Anne and loves to spend long hours working in the garden. Above all, she plans to remain a 'with it'' mother and grandmother to her loving family.

Fred Hennigan 82

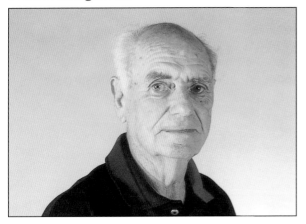

Fred began practicing yoga when he turned 80! He attends regular weekly classes with his wife Lorna. Together they have found yoga has for them, reversed the aging process. They feel more energetic, more flexible and capable of looking after their own house and garden. Fred is always happy to modify any practices to suit his own level of strength and flexibility. Fred enjoys all the yoga practices including the standing poses and the relaxation and meditation practices.

Lorna Hennigan 74

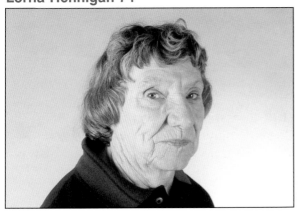

When Lorna began yoga classes 3 years ago, she had bad arthritis and was very stiff in her hips. Over the last few years, Lorna's arthritis is much improved. Her mobility everywhere, especially in the hips, has given her a new sense of freedom knowing that getting older doesn't mean physical deterioration. New levels of energy have seen Lorna learn to swim and go back to her love of singing. Lorna enjoys the company of her husband Fred and the other class members and has made many new friendships.

Louise Wiggins 55

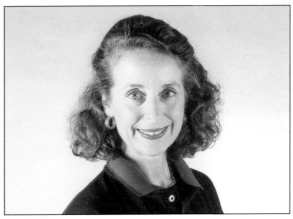

Like many of my students, I turned to yoga as a result of feeling unwell. Abdominal surgery, arthritis, sciatica, lack of energy, persistent bladder infection were just some of the reasons I looked for an intelligent system of caring for myself . I wanted to take full responsibility for my own well being and found all the answers in yoga. I feel better now than ever before. Each day I thank yoga for its precious gift of energy, stillness, harmony, strength, flexibility and a holistic sense of well being.

Growing a Younger Body

Section2 Section2 Section

Asanas, The Postures: Moving it or losing it

Eastern Legend: The Frog in the Well
There once was a small frog, who lived in a well. He was born in this well and knew no other world. One day, another frog who came from the sea, fell into the well. The well frog asked the sea frog where he came from and the sea frog said that he came from the sea. "How big is the sea?" asked the well frog. "It is very big." said the sea frog. Asked how big the sea was, the sea frog said, "Very, very big." The frog in the well stretched out his arms and legs and said, "This big?" "Much, much bigger than that," replied the frog from the sea. "Is it as big as this well?" asked the well frog. "My dear friend, it is impossible to compare this small well with the vast sea." At this the small frog became very angry. "Nothing could ever be as big as this well. You are a liar and you had better leave at once." said the narrow minded frog, unable to conceive of a larger world than his own small well.

So let's begin our practice with the wide open mind.
In the pages that follow, you'll find yoga postures selected to help mobilise all the joints in the body, to stimulate circulation and to stretch and strengthen all the major muscle groups. You'll soon find that the strength and flexibility obtained is much more than just physical.

Before you begin
Before beginning any fitness program, please consult your health professional if you have any doubts about your ability to exercise, at this time.

Be ultimately in tune with your body's own natural intelligence so that you know just how far to proceed in any of the yoga practices.

Before You Begin: Helpful Hints and Cautions

Before you begin, take a few moments to read through these cautions and hints for a safe yoga practice, always remembering to honour your unique body as it is, not expecting too much and allowing it to unfold in its own time.

I allow my body to unfold and blossom in its own time, like a rose bud to a bloom.

- Yoga is non competitive.

- Yoga is your own unique experience of the practice.

- Let your practice unfold from within.

- Yoga is a holistic approach to your well being.

- Always work within the limits of your own abilities.

- Never strain, but also, don't limit yourself.

- Pain is a warning sign to stop or modify your practice.

- Learn the difference between pain and the exquisite sensation of an intense stretch.

- Never use force. Be gentle with yourself.

- Never hold the breath, let it flow freely.

- Wear loose, comfortable clothing.

- Practice with bare feet on a safe, non-slip surface.

- In forward bends, keep the spine long and straight, bending at the hip with the knees soft and torso fully supported.

- Don't restrict your airways. Keep the chest open, shoulders relaxed. It will help asthma sufferers gain relief.

- Be satisfied with small improvements in your mobility.

- With high blood pressure, heart problems, detached retina, glaucoma, avoid inverted postures where the head is lower than the heart.

- Relax into the postures as you exhale. Your body's natural wisdom will guide you.

- Allow each exhalation to take you deeper into your body.

- Breathe freely in and out of the nostrils at all times.

- Allow 3-4 hours after main meals and 1-2 hours after snacks, before exercise.

- Arms too short? Legs too long? Use a belt or strap.

- Work slowly, letting your body unfold when it's ready. Give it your full attention.

- Dizziness is a sign to stop and relax for a few minutes.

- Listen to your body and heed its advice.

- Enjoy your yoga practice. Have fun. Smile and do it now!

- Don't forget that the body whispers and talks to us before it screams. Listen to the whispers!

Growing Younger

Incontinence

Incontinence is the lack of control over bladder and bowel movement. We are born incontinent and as we age, this problem has a tendency to return!
In women, the uterus and pelvic floor tends to sag as we grow older.
Pelvic floor exercises can really help to restore muscle tone. Find which muscles to strengthen by stopping your urine flow midstream. Then during the day, at any time, contract those muscles often! Promise yourself 100 contractions a day and see the amazing difference that can make.

   So find the right muscles, then contract, hold for a moment, relax and repeat 100 times. Include it in your yoga posture practice. Try it while in the inverted postures.

Mountain Pose Tadasana

Growing a younger posture

The upright standing position called mountain pose, is one of yoga's most important poses. Whenever you stand, gently focus your attention on this pose for better posture and a more efficient functioning of the glands and organs of the body.

Standing Still, Standing Firm

Stand with the body evenly balanced on both feet and feeling the weight of the body evenly distributed on the soles of the feet. Feet pointing straight ahead. Press gently with the big toes to lift the arches. Feel the energy moving upwards as the weight of your body moves downwards, feeling grounded and secure. Visualise that there is a cord that extends from the crown of the head to the ceiling and that your body is lengthening upwards along this cord. Experience the spaciousness along the spine, shoulder girdle and neck area.

Grounded and Growing

Allow the spine to elongate, the neck to lengthen, the face to soften, the weight to be evenly distributed on both feet. Allow the shoulders to move up back and down. Kneecaps lifted, knees unlocked. Experience the spine comfortable in its natural curves. Take a moment to allow the breath to gently deepen into the solar plexus, your still calm centre, like the ground level of a plant. Allow each exhalation to flow down and up simultaneously, creating a sensation of spaciousness from the hara centre up to the crown of the head and from the hara centre down to the soles of the feet. Feeling grounded and growing at the same time.

Experience the upward flow of energy from your hara centre to the crown of the head, the shoulders and down both arms all the way to the fingertips. Experience the downward flow from the hara centre to the pelvis and down both legs all the way down to the soles of the feet. Grounded and growing. Standing still and standing firm.

Helpful Hint

You may like to check your alignment in Mountain Pose by using a pendulum, strap, or lead line. Place one end at the hip joint and look down to see if the bottom of the pendulum hangs beside the ankle. Most people find that they need to move the pelvis back about 10cm. Notice how this little shift, creates new space in the lumbar back.

Growing upwards towards the light

Hara centre

Centred in stillness

Growing down, grounding, standing firm, anchored and secure

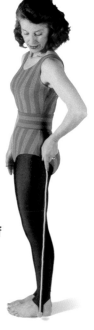

Check your posture with a pendulum.

Warming Up

Taking the time to prepare the body for safe practice.
Here are some warm up postures to practice on the floor so that there is least strain on your spine. It is important to carefully warm the body before you begin your practice. Enrich your experience of the movements by allowing them to flow in harmony with your free flowing breath.

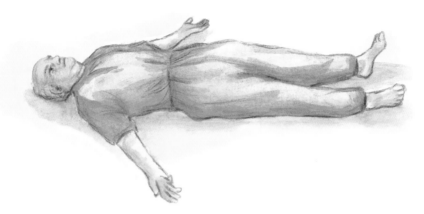

Relaxation Pose
Always begin your practice in relaxation pose so that you have a few moments to tune into your body's needs. The blood flow is equalised, muscles relax, organs rejuvenate as the mind quietens. See p96 for more details.

Full Body Stretch
Stretch the arms beyond the head in two straight lines allowing the back of the hands to touch the floor behind, all 10 fingernails on the floor if you can. Rotate the feet to warm the ankles and stimulate the circulation.

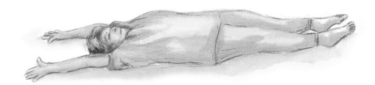

Stretching the Back of the Spine
Gently hug the knees to the chest and bring the nose towards the knees as far as you're comfortable. Stay there for several breaths allowing the spine to lengthen in its own time.

Stretching the Front of the Spine.
With the knees bent and in line with the hips, gently lift the buttocks off the floor until you feel a comfortable stretch sensation along the front of the whole spine. Gently pinch the buttocks muscles together, scooping the pelvis up to lengthen the lumbar back.

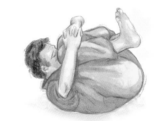

Twisting the Spine

With the feet wider than the hips, allow the low back to settle against the floor. When you're ready, allow the knees to fall to the right and the head to the left. Bring the knees back to centre and allow the knees to fall to the left, head right. Continue this movement in harmony with your breath. Inhaling knees coming up, exhaling, knees falling to one side. Do an even number on each side.

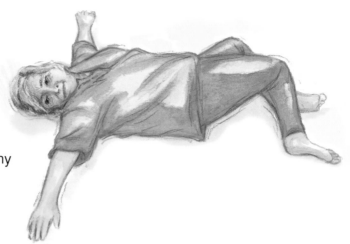

Stretching the Hamstrings

With a tie or strap around the sole of the foot, allow the back of the leg to lengthen to benefit the hip joint as well as the knee joint. You'll get most benefit from the stretch if you allow the back of the knee to open and the breath to flow freely. Notice how each exhalation allows you to move a little further along the ceiling. Experience the breath. Each inhalation energises the whole leg as you feel the foot press into the strap. Experience a release of tightness and contraction with each exhalation.

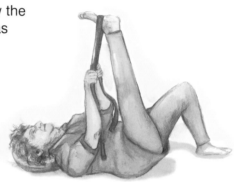

Opening the Hips

Bend the knee and hold the foot with both hands, gently drawing the heel towards the navel and rocking the leg from side to side.

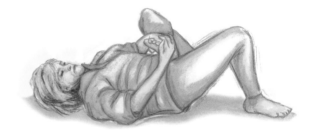

Hips, Knees and Ankles

Bring the soles of the feet together and hold the ankles or feet. Stay there for several breaths allowing the joints to respond when they're ready. Check that the back of the neck is still long and relaxed. Smile! Let your body open to the stretch.

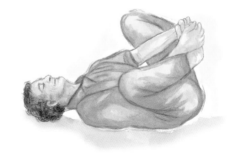

Growing Younger

Airflow
Good muscle tone in the abdomen will help to create an even, smooth, comfortable air flow through the body. Prana, life force and energy are then delivered to all the cells in the body using the breath as its mode of transportation.
Receive the energy with each inhalation. Let go of any tension with each exhalation.

Massage the Back
With the knees hugged to the chest, roll from side to side to massage the low back, back of the waist and shoulder girdle. Enjoy the sensation of the long erector muscles along the spine being massaged.

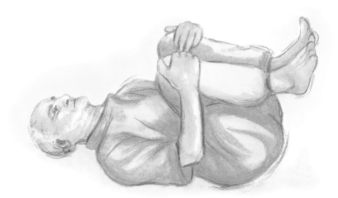

Snuggling on the Side
Roll over onto the right side away from the heart and stay snuggled up in this fetal position for a few moments, whole body soft and relaxed.

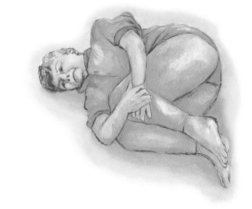

Stretching the Shoulders and Back
Coming up onto all fours. Walk the hands about 2 hand lengths further forward. Now lower your body towards the floor as far as it comfortably can. Let the spine stretch and lengthen. Let the shoulder girdle open and release. Experience the exquisite release of tension along the whole spine and across the shoulders with every breath out.

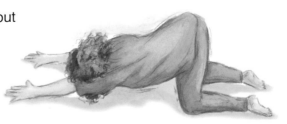

Inversions

Turning back the clock, keeping you young.
Inverted postures are even more important to do every day as we get older. They are our anti-gravity and anti-wrinkle poses helping us to win the war against sagging skin and prolapsing organs.

Growing Younger

The benefits of inverted postures
Inverted postures increase the blood flow to the brain (we have more than a 100 billion neurons!) to benefit every vital organ in the head including the pituitary gland thereby increasing mental and physical efficiency. Digestion is improved as well as relieving constipation and prolapse problems. The whole endocrine system benefits and is reflected in the whole body.

Gravity
The force of gravity is the strongest force acting on our body. It shapes our body and literally drags us down. Jumping and climbing soon reminds us of how true that is!

Gravity acts on our body fluids, as liquid in a vessel. It drops down. Blood pools in the legs as we stand and drains from the brain and vital organs.

The Heart
The venous blood circulation propels the blood up against the force of gravity. It stands to reason that when we lie down, the heart can rest.

When we invert the body the benefits are even greater as the venous blood returns effortlessly back to the heart. So you can see the importance of inversions. They rest the heart, restore tone in the vital organs, rejuvenate the brain, as they relieve varicose veins. No wonder we feel refreshed and rejuvenated whenever we take the time to invert the whole body.

Taking Care
With blood pressure problems, glaucoma and heart conditions, it is not advisable to lower the head below the heart, so seek medical advice before beginning any exercise program. But don't give up! You can invert the lower half of the body. Try the first two practices. Never strain or hold your breath.

The Shoulder Stand
Begin with the legs up the wall. Bend the knees, push the feet into the wall until the buttocks lift off. Support the hands under the hips and rise higher if you're comfortable. Tuck the elbows in so that they are approximately in line with the shoulders.

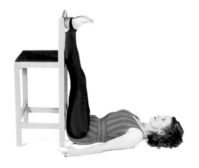

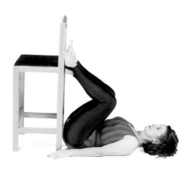

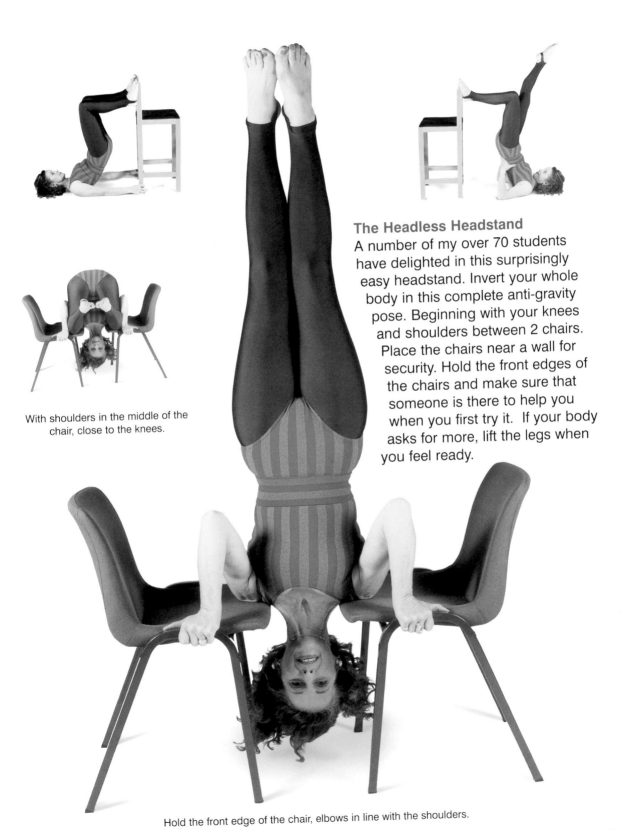

With shoulders in the middle of the chair, close to the knees.

The Headless Headstand

A number of my over 70 students have delighted in this surprisingly easy headstand. Invert your whole body in this complete anti-gravity pose. Beginning with your knees and shoulders between 2 chairs. Place the chairs near a wall for security. Hold the front edges of the chairs and make sure that someone is there to help you when you first try it. If your body asks for more, lift the legs when you feel ready.

Hold the front edge of the chair, elbows in line with the shoulders.

Looking For Opportunities to Invert Every Day

Make a resolve that you will invert your body every single day from now on, for the rest of your life! Below are just some of the ways to invert your body each day. Have fun and experience the benefits.

Legs On a Chair
To rest the back, and ease tired legs

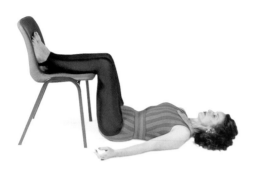

Legs Up the Wall
For tired legs, varicose veins and swollen ankles. It feel so good, you'll want to stay there forever!

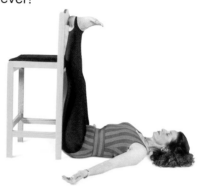

Ironing Board Slope
The best ever use for your ironing board! A complete gentle inversion to ease prolapse of bladder, bowel and uterus. Varicose veins drain as you rejuvenate the whole body and all its vital organs. Contract the muscles of the pelvic floor to benefit both prolapse and incontinence. Please see 'Taking Care' on the previous page before you proceed.

I will invert my body every day for the rest of my life.

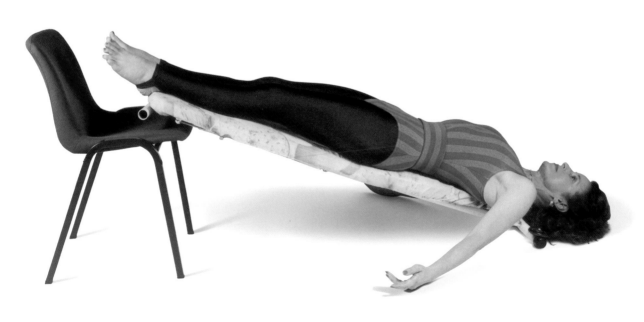

Play Ball

Lie down on the floor with the knees bent, feet flat. Push the feet into the floor to lift the buttocks, then slip the ball (a cheap plastic football works really well) under the buttocks and allow the legs to drift up towards the ceiling keeping the knees soft.

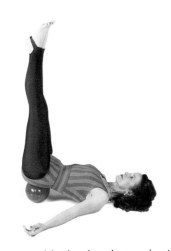

Half Handstand

Feel like a child again as you strengthen the arms. Begin in dog pose with the heels against the wall. Then slowly begin to walk up the wall. Take care not to collapse in the shoulders. Experience the strength. Push with the roots of your fingers. Wrists sore? See p63. Caution: see 'taking care' p56.

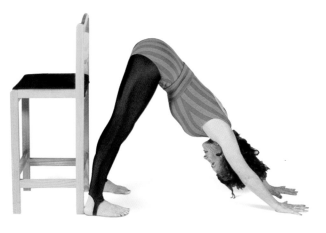

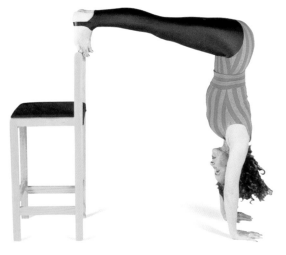

Yoga teaches

that there are no limitations to what we can achieve if we know and understand the power of the breath when it creates a free flow of energy through the body and the mind. There are no limitations when we combine this power with the power of the asanas (yoga poses) and the creative power of the mind.

Mental health

Prolong your mental health by listening to your body's natural intelligence when choosing treatment, buying food, and any other lifestyle choices. Each cell in your body is constantly renewing, healing and replacing itself. The stretching, relaxation and breathing practices of yoga will help you maintain an exquisite natural mental and physical balance.

Triangle Pose Trikonasana

Strength and flexibility for the whole body

Triangle pose gives the whole body a complete stretch with special benefits for the shoulders, chest, legs, spine and the spinal nerves. You'll find it a pose to uplift, enliven and invigorate you as it benefits the whole nervous system and stimulates all your body's organs and joints. Take care to progress slowly and let your body unfold in its own time.

Preparation

Step your feet wide apart to make an equilateral (or a little wider) triangle with your legs. Arms at shoulder height, fingers extended. Turn the right foot out and the left foot in. Lift the kneecaps, feeling the strength rising up the legs along the spine and into the arms and fingers with each inhalation.

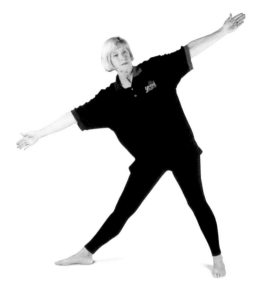

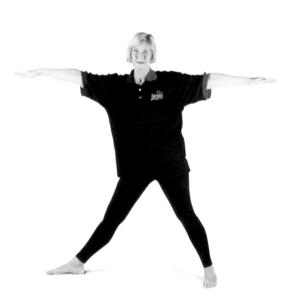

Half Triangle

Hold your leg there. Wait for your body to open with your breath and you may find you can go a little further into the pose. Never strain or hold the breath. Smile!

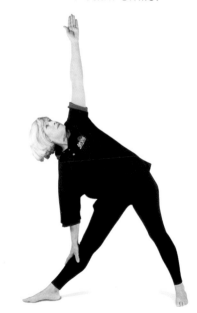

Feel the Window

Imagine that there is a large window pane right in front of you. Turn the palms forwards to face the 'window'. Spread the fingers and move the arms like a windmill to sense where the 'window' is, without touching or crashing through it. Now allow the right fingers to touch the right leg, the left fingers reaching up. Breathe spaciousness into the joints.

Full Triangle Pose

When you're ready, explore how far you can comfortably proceed towards full triangle, without breaking the 'window'. Reach for your best potential. Repeat on the other side.

Counter Pose

The Waterfall Uttanasana
Place your hands on the thighs, knees or shins. Allow the spine to lengthen as it cascades forward. Also p52 and p56 for cautions: 'taking care'.

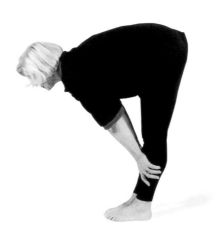

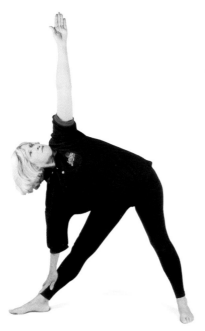

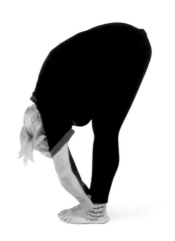

Taking It Gently

When Joyce couldn't bear weight on her foot, she practiced triangle pose using a chair.

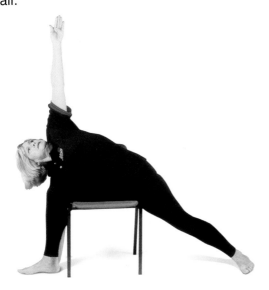

Growing Younger

Relief from back pain
90% of spinal discomfort in the form of aches and pains can be relieved by the practice of regular, gentle yoga stretches, performed in harmony with the breath and giving them your full attention.

Dog Pose Adho Mukha Svanasana

This is an all-in-one posture. Make a resolve to do the DOG every day. Dog pose promotes upper body strength, as it flattens the upper back. It is a comfortable inversion and is sometimes called the gentle version of the yoga headstand. It straightens and strengthens the spine and stretches the backs of the legs. It energises your whole being as it rests the heart and allows you to breathe deeply. It helps with prolapse problems as it strengthens the joints and relieves arthritis in the shoulders.
Experience the exhilaration of dog pose for yourself.

Back of the Chair Dog
To lengthen the spine and open the shoulders. Make sure that the chair is braced against the wall for safe practice. Focus on elongating the spine, navel drawn in and the arms and legs in line with the shoulders and hips. If this is comfortable, try the next pose.

Seat of the Chair Dog
To deepen the shoulder stretch. Align the arms and legs as before, experience a deeper stretch along the spine, shoulders and backs of the legs. Let the breath open your body to the full.

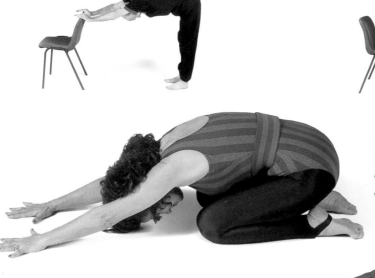

Dog Pose
Here's how to allow this gentle version of the yoga headstand to work its magic on you.

Begin on all fours, sitting back towards the heels arms stretched beyond the head in two straight parallel lines.

When you're ready, curl the toes under and straighten the legs a little, keeping the spine flat and the navel drawn in to support the low back. Bend the knees as much as you need to, to straighten the spine and stretch across the shoulders.

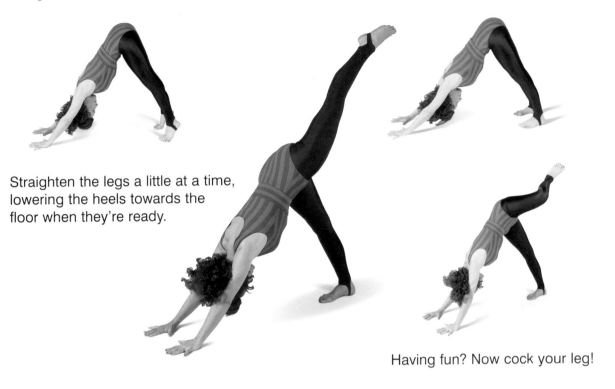

Straighten the legs a little at a time, lowering the heels towards the floor when they're ready.

Having fun? Now cock your leg!

Wrists Uncomfortable?
Move the weight onto the roots of the fingers, but if you are still uncomfortable try these modifications.

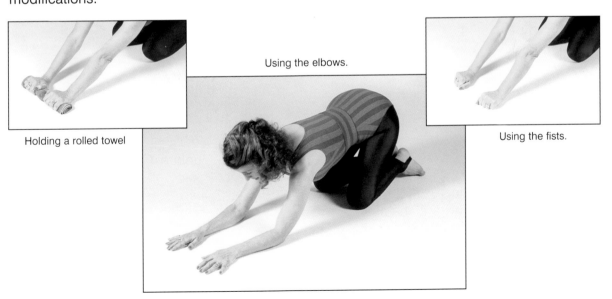

Using the elbows.

Holding a rolled towel

Using the fists.

Strength

Keeping bones and muscles young

As we age, we tend to lose muscle tissue. To maintain strong bones, we need strong muscles to pull and tug on the skeleton to prevent bones from weakening. As we lose bone tissue, we begin to develop osteoporosis. So keep strong and active.

Try some of these poses and surprise yourself. You'll feel wonderfully invigorated and totally alive!

Hands, Arms and Wrists

1. Push ups face down

Lying on the front of your body, with the hands under the shoulders, elbows tucked in and the knees bent. Pinch the buttocks, draw the navel in and push up, breathing strength into the arms.

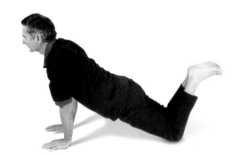

2. Push ups face up

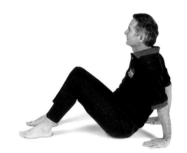

(i) Sit with the knees bent at 90 degrees and the hands behind you, shoulder width apart.

(ii) If you're comfortable, push up making a table while keeping the neck long and shoulders drawn away from the ears. Try to keep the knees in line with the hips.

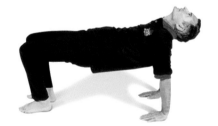

(iii) Sit between the hands in rod posture. Repeat these last 3 movements several more times.

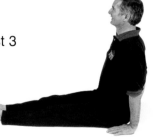

3. Arm Balance Vasisthasana

Try plank pose. Begin by supporting your body on your hands and toes. Tuck the tail under to lengthen the lumbar back. Draw the navel in towards the spine for strength and support.

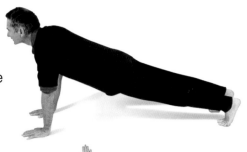

Now roll to one side and push! Smile! Arm turning to jelly?! Breathe into the heart and send strength into the supporting arm as you exhale. It really works! Repeat on the other side.

My body and my mind are strong and flexible.

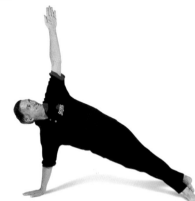

Yoga teaches
Yoga teaches the body, mind and breath are one with the universe. You will soon notice that the strength and flexibility of the body are reflected in the mind.

Helpful Hints
• Many people find that when they first try to bear weight on their arms, the arms turn to jelly!
• Experience the difference when you breathe deeply into the heart and as you exhale direct a flow of strength into the supporting limb.
• Allow the strength to flow from within
• Don't collapse in the shoulders, maintain a sensation of spaciousness and support

Having Trouble Balancing?
• Press all the toes into the floor, allowing the arches to lift.
• Stand near a wall or hold a chair.
• Focus your gaze on the floor ahead of you and steady your mind as you slow the breath.
• Lengthen the tail bone towards the heels, soften the knees, with the abdomen slightly drawn in.
• Lengthen the back of the neck, positioning the ears directly over the shoulders.
• Keep the breath flowing freely.
• Feel grounded, centred, alive.

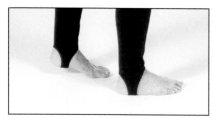

Toes, Feet and Ankles

The best way to strengthen the feet and the toes is to walk barefoot on the beach at the water's edge. letting the sea and sand massage the soles of the feet and improving circulation. So take off your shoes and experience your feet!

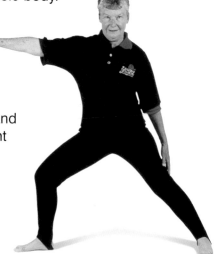

Coming up on the toes

With the toes, ankles and knees pressed firmly together, slowly rise up on the toes. Stay in this position for several more breaths. Keep the ankles together! Experience the strength in the feet.

I am grounded in strength and resolve. I stand firm.

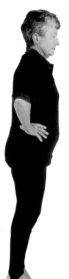

The Chair Pose

Slowly bend the knees and sit on an imaginary chair. Keep the toes, ankles and knees pressed together. Experience the strength in the legs and abdomen. Extend the arms to shoulder height and stay there for several breaths.

Whole Body

The Warrior Pose helps you to strengthen the muscles, bones and joints of the whole body.

Warrior Pose Virabhadrasana II
Warrior Pose Preparation

Spread the legs wide apart with the right foot turned out and the left foot turned in. Rest the left hand near the knee joint with the right hand extended at shoulder height. Look along the right arm. Bend the right knee as near to 90 degrees as you comfortably can, keeping the knee directly over the ankle. Allow the left hand to slide a little more towards the back knee. Feeling upright and strong.

Warrior Pose
When you're ready, extend both arms to shoulder height and sink down into the strength of warrior pose. Experience the stillness within the strength. Take a moment to allow yourself to experience the strength deepening.

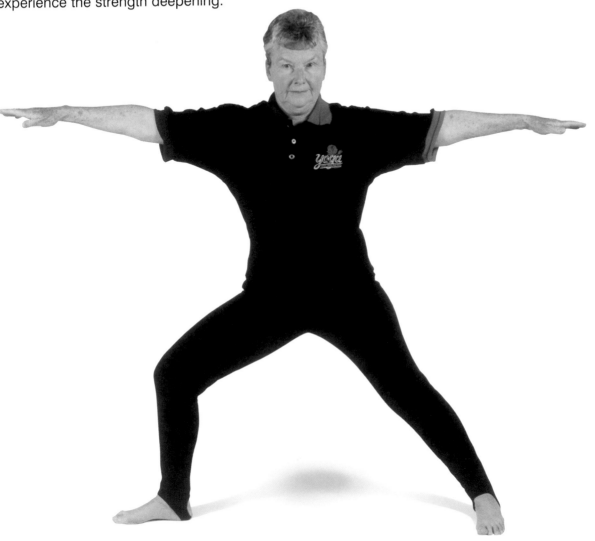

I rest in the stillness of my inner strength

Today I will open the door to my calmness,
And let the footsteps of silence gently enter the temple of all my activities.
I will perform my duties serenely, saturated with peace.
(Yogananda)

Flexibility

Keeping the joints and organs young
Flexibility is life. Stiffness is death. The slang word for a corpse is in fact a 'stiff'! We can see this truth all around us.

The Toa teaches us that a young tree is flexible, whereas an old tree is stiff.
When we are born, we are flexible. When we die we are stiff.
A flexible body will give us a flexible mind so that we can continue to grow and evolve, happy and receptive to new ideas.

1. Hands, Wrists and Elbows
Practice this easy flowing sequence often.
Begin with the palms together, whole hand touching whole hand, with the thumbs at the notch in the sternum, feeling centred and ready.

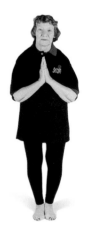

Allow the thumbs to descend to the heart level, allowing the inner wrists to stretch.

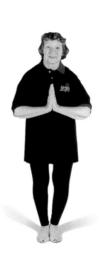

Now open the hands like a book.

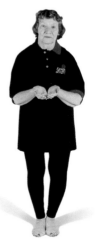

Roll the back of the hands together, fingers now pointing towards you.

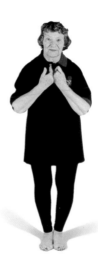

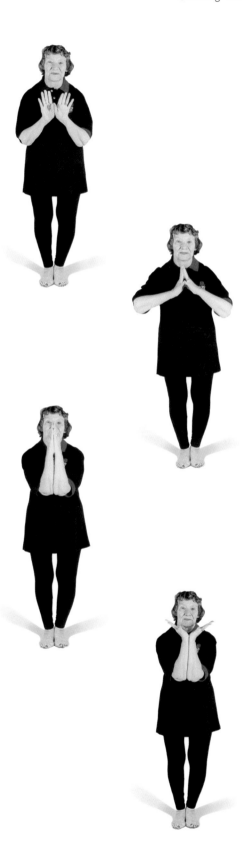

Bring the thumbs together, palms facing out before coming back to the starting position, palms facing.

Press the tips of the fingers together making a triangle with your hands. Spread the fingers as wide as comfortable before allowing them to lower down slowly towards the navel or even the pubis, giving the fingers and wrists a vigorous backbend, keeping them flexible and supple.

Bring the hands back to the sternum and allow them to rise towards the ceiling, higher and higher, keeping the elbows together.

When the elbows are at shoulder height, allow the fingertips to open and spread like a blossoming flower. Space all the fingers evenly around your 'flower'.

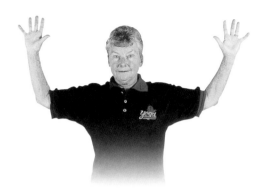

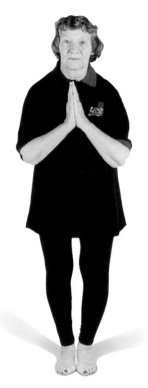

Now stretch the right arm up. Lower the shoulder and let the arm move back as far as comfortable.

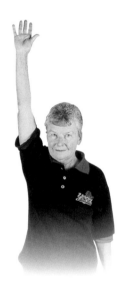

Come back to the starting position and repeat the whole sequence 4 more times.

Yoga teaches

Yoga teaches that when the backbone stiffens, old age begins. A flexible spine will allow a free circulation of life force to all the body's joints and organs to nourish, cleanse and rejuvenate every cell.

2. Arms and Shoulders

With the elbows bent, palms facing forward and hands at shoulder level, visualise that there is a pane of glass and your palms are on the glass. Now make small movements, 'washing' the window near your palms. Reverse the direction when you're ready. Experience the small movements in the arms and the shoulders for the prevention and relief of 'frozen shoulders'.

Growing Younger

Arthritis

Yoga teaches that the mind and the breath are our most powerful medicine and available at any time for no cost. With a quiet mind and a free flowing breath, yoga will stretch and mobilise all the joints to suit your own unique individual needs. Yoga practices will take your joints and give them a general service. Arthritic joints will be nourished and nurtured and will be less painful.

When you're ready bend the elbow and give yourself a well deserved pat on the back, right between the shoulder blades. If you're comfortable and your body asks for more, hold bent the elbow with the other hand to give yourself a further stretch. Hold and breathe.

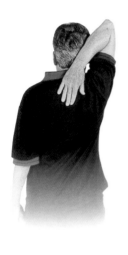
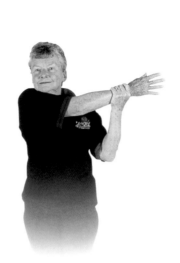
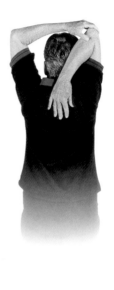

When you're ready, straighten the arm under the chin, holding the wrist with the opposite hand and lengthening the arm, opening the right shoulder joint and upper back. Repeat the last 3 movements with the left arm.

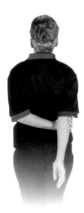
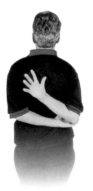

Hold the right elbow with your left hand behind the back. 'Breathe' the right shoulder blade down and towards the centre of the spine. Hold for a moment while you breathe evenly and smoothly.

If you would like a further stretch, bend the right arm and hold the elbow allowing the back of the right hand to move towards the space between the shoulder blades. Repeat with the left arm.

Cow Face Posture
Gomukasana

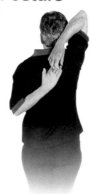

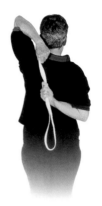

Put these 2 practices together and try the cow face pose.

Use a strap, tie or belt to 'lengthen' your arms! Don't be a coward, and cower, smile!

Growing Younger

Helpful Hint

Cow Face posture is challenging, but don't give up. Do the best you can, knowing the benefits of flexibility in the shoulder girdle. Gently, and in its own time, allow stiff joints to open within your comfort zone, when they're ready. All you have to do is breathe and wait patiently, holding the pose for several breaths.

---

3. Toes and Feet

Four times around the world
Consider your amazing feet.
It is estimated that during a lifetime we walk around the earth about 4 times! Feet are the foundation of your mobility, so take good care of them. These little platforms have to bare the weight of your whole body.

Footwear

Study your footwear and consider whether they may be responsible for any pain you may experience. Do your socks and shoes allow full movement, yet adequate support? Are your shoes really the right size? See a foot specialist if you have any doubts. Orthotics can work wonders for feet, hips, spine and whole body imbalances as well as fallen arches.

You have 26 bones in the feet. These need correct alignment and adequate space to serve you well. Allow your feet to experience the prickly grass, the grainy sand and the soft carpet. Spread your toes at every opportunity. So take off your shoes and stretch the toes. Here are some healthy yoga feet and toes.

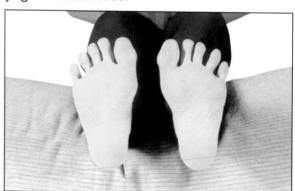

Using the fingers to put space between the toes. Hold, breathe, and slowly begin to circle the toes, in both directions holding the top and sole of the foot with the other hand. When you're finished, experience the warmth in the foot before doing the other one.

Straighten the big toes, using a ponytailer. Spread the little ones using your fingers. Your toes will love this stretch.

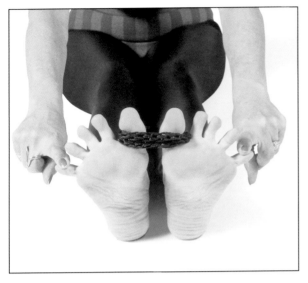 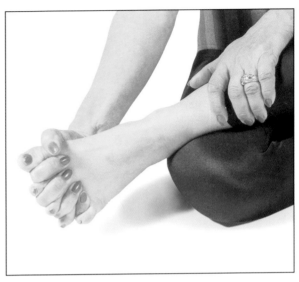

4. Knees and Hips

Open the knees and hip joints as you stretch the hamstrings for a healthier back. The knees too benefit, as the hamstrings cross the knee joints, as well as the hip joints.

Healthy hamstrings for healthy knees and back
Lying down in the semi-supine position with the neck long, shoulders relaxed, face soft. Place a strap or tie, over the sole of the right foot and straighten the leg as much as comfortable. Experience the stretch behind the knee as you open the back of the leg more with each exhalation. Take a moment to experience your best stretch position. Allow the breath to flow into the area of stretch and let go more and more with each breath.

When you're ready, bend the knee, drawing the heel towards the navel and rock the leg from side to side. Place the foot on your heart! Place the big toe on your forehead! Smile.

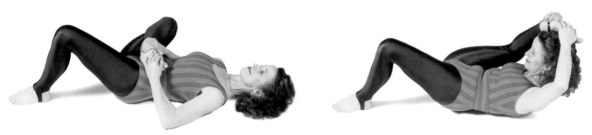

I am calm and relaxed.
My breath is a free flow of energy rippling through my body's organs and joints.

Growing Younger

Young feet

Have you looked at your feet lately? Do you notice any imbalance? Perhaps they don't look the same, or their alignment in uneven. Check for any differences. Check for any stiffness. You may find that a visit to the foot specialist will help to correct this imbalance. Orthotics have been most helpful in alleviating foot, back and neck problems.

5. The Spine

The spine loves it when you twist it from the base of the spine right up into the neck. A healthy, flexible spine will not only make you feel wonderful, it allows you the freedom to do what you want painlessly and effortlessly. See the 'Spine Savers' on page 112-115 for a complete workout.

Here is a little sequence your spine will love.

1. Head to Knee Pose janu sirsanasa

Sitting on a cushion if your hamstrings are tight, take a moment to elongate the front of the spine. You'll feel yourself rolling onto the front of the sitting bones. Bend the right leg and draw the foot into the inner thigh or knee. Keeping the spine long and looking up, draw the navel in and lengthen over the leg using a strap if you need one.

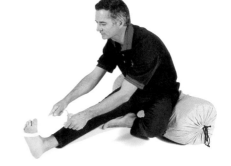

2. Twist and turn

With the spine still straight and long, take the left hand to the right knee and twist the spine from its base to the crown of the head. Allow the spine to lengthen with each inhalation. Allow the spine to twist a little further with each exhalation. Lengthen the back of the neck, chin tucked in a little, to allow you to twist deeper into the neck and shoulder girdle.

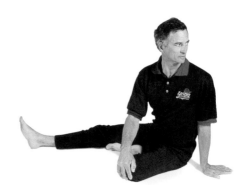

3. Side stretch

Come back to centre. With the left hand on the bent right knee, stretch the right arm alongside the ear, reaching up with your in-breath, and gently stretching to the side with your out-breath. Experience an exquisite opening of the side ribs and spine.

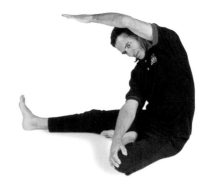

Strong bones
Keep your bones strong by including more calcium rich foods in your daily diet. Be sure to include low fat dairy products, yogurt, fish with bones (sardines, salmon) almonds, calcium enriched soy milk, tahini (a delicious paste made from sesame seeds) and lots of dark green vegetables. Look for products fortified with calcium.

See P98-99 for some delicious healthy food ideas.

> ## Yoga teaches
> Yoga teaches that the health of the spine reflects the health of the whole body.

4. Stretching up
Taking your weight on the right arm behind you, reach for the ceiling with your left hand. When you're ready, push your buttocks off the floor and reach for your best potential.

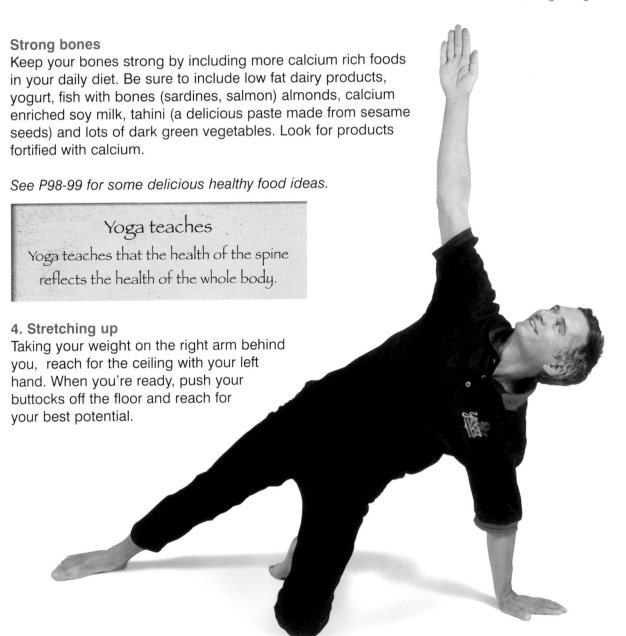

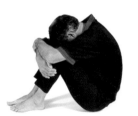

5. Release and surrender
Bring the knees together, give yourself a big hug and allow the eyeballs to rest on the knees. Allow the spine, shoulders, neck to soften and release. Now you're ready to repeat 1-5 with the left leg.

My breath is the bridge between my body and my mind.

Balancing

Standing on your own two feet. Keeping you grounded and centred
Yoga offers the gift of balance and harmony between all the different aspects of ourselves. As you begin to find this harmony, you'll find balances become easier. As you practice the balancing poses, notice the constant adjustments you need to make. Allow these adjustments to remind you to be physically , emotionally and mentally flexible and willing to change.

Sitting Balances
These sitting balances will help strengthen the abdominal muscles as they strengthen the legs. Take your time and do just as much as you can.

The Boat pose Navasana
Sit upright, spine long, shoulders relaxed, knees bent, holding the backs of the thighs. On your exhalation, draw the navel in and experience your abdominal strength.

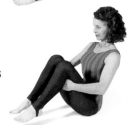

When you're ready, continue to elongate the spine, lift the feet and balance on the sitting bones. Lengthen the space between the pubis and the sternum.

Straighten the legs as much as you can to experience the boat pose. Smile. Listen to the wisdom of your body to guide you to your best position.

Don't sink your ship; be sea worthy.
This pose is not called the Titanic!

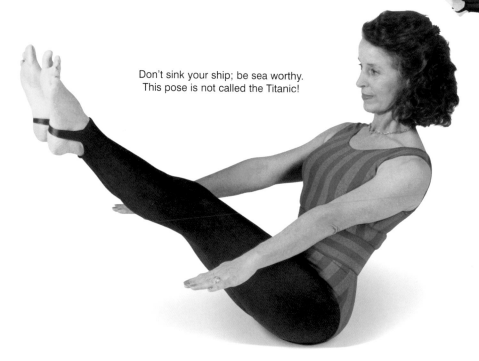

Standing Balance

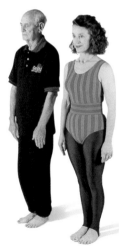

Tree Pose Vrksasana

These 2 poses are called tree balances. They help you to feel grounded, balanced, centred and alive. Growing upwards towards the light yet strong, flexible and grounded, in perfect harmony with the natural balance in nature. You're now ready to do the other side.

I am centred and focussed, grounded and growing. My life is unfolding just as it should.

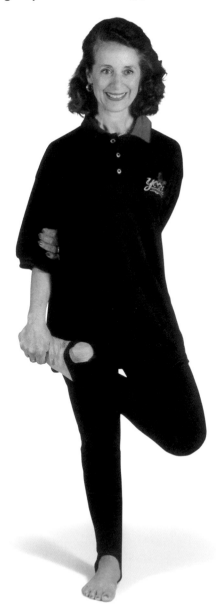

Always begin your standing postures in Mountain pose. Transfer the weight onto the right foot and position the left foot on the right instep, knee or inner thigh to suit your own flexibility at this time.
Bring the palms of the hands together at the centre of the chest and observe the breath. Breathe energy into the abdomen on the inhalation. When you're ready to exhale, radiate the energy down and up simultaneously.

Now try holding the left foot with the right hand, whilst holding the right elbow with the left hand behind the back.

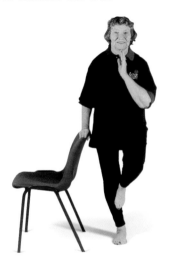

Back Bends

Stopping the spine rounding by stretching the front of the spine, while bending over backwards for a healthier back and better breathing. If you were asked to act really old, what would you do? You'd probably round your shoulders and stoop forward! As we get older, we tend to lose muscle tissue, lose strength and find that we grow shorter as the spine begins to round and compress.

It becomes even more important to continue to practice backbends, to open the chest and strengthen the spine.

Youthful Posture

When the spine rounds forward, the shoulders round and the chest collapses. This restricts breathing. The cells receive limited oxygen supplies leading to health and heart problems. So be conscious of maintaining a youthful upright posture to allow the inner organs and the nervous system to function at optimum levels.

Crocodile Pose Makarasana

Lying on the front of your body with the forehead resting on the back of your hands. Relax the spine and shoulder girdle. This is an excellent pose for observing your deep diaphragmatic breath.

Half Locust Pose

Tuck the arms alongside the body, palms down under the hips, elbows tucked in. Lengthen your tail and draw the navel towards the spine. Inhale, exhale, lift the right leg, keeping the hips down. Do the other side. Repeat 5 times on each side.

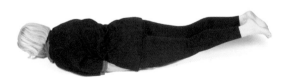

Full Locust Pose Salabhasana

With the arms as before, inhale, exhale and lift both legs as high as comfortable. Hold the position if you can while you allow the breath to flow freely. Experience the strength in the back muscles.

Sphinx Pose
With the elbows under the shoulders, neck long, shoulders down, relax the spine. Lengthen the back of the neck.

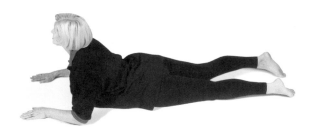

Release in Swan Pose
Bring the buttocks towards the heels, arms stretched overhead and in line with the shoulders. Release and allow the heart to sink down towards the floor. Experience the whole spine, long and relaxed.

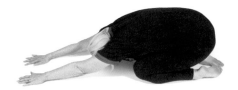

As I breathe in, I breathe in healing energy.
As I breathe out, I smile.

Growing Younger

Helpful Hints and Cautions

- Keep the belly soft.
- When standing, allow the low back to lengthen by softening the knees, keeping them lightly bent.
- Keep the breath freely flowing.
- Lengthen the back of the neck by lifting the base of the skull away from the shoulders.
- Gently pinch the buttock muscles together and draw in the lower abdomen to support the lumbar spine and tilt the pelvis.
- Allow the shoulders to move up, back and down.
- Listen to your body. If your low back complains, you may have stretched too far.
- Smile.

Yoga teaches
We are as young as the spine is flexible.
Old age begins when we allow the spine to stiffen.

Forward Bends

Giving the whole back of the body an intense stretch.
Forward bends are challenging and will help to develop perseverance because we will often be putting ourselves in a situation where we're not comfortable and want to hurry. But don't give up. Forward bends massage and stimulate the inner organs as you stretch and energise the spine. Be patient with yourself. Simply breathe into your best extension.

Take Your Time

It is well worth the effort to take your time to practice forward bends safely. Before you try the following poses, look at Colleen's demonstration of how to proceed. Always elongate the spine first. Think of lengthening the space between the pubis and the sternum, adding a couple more millimetres with each inhalation and bending further forward a couple of millimetres with each exhalation.

Sitting Forward Bend
Full forward bend paschimottanasa
Use a strap to lengthen your arms so that you can keep the spine elongating. Simply breathe and wait for your body to unfold and ask you for more stretch. Enjoy the sensations you experience.
Another way to practice is to bend the knees and rest the abdomen on the thighs to support the lumbar spine.

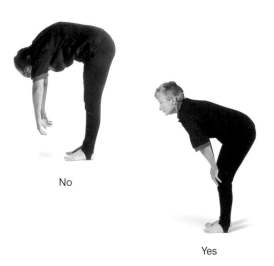

No

Yes

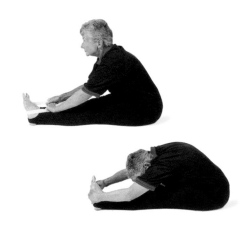

Kneeling Forward Bend
Child pose pranatasana

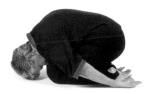

Allow the spine to lengthen safely with the low back supported by the thighs.

Standing Forward Bend
Touching the toes uttanasana
Don't forget to lengthen the spine and support the weight of the torso so that you don't strain your back. To come up again, bend your knees, tuck the chin in, draw the navel in and uncurl bringing the head up last.

Notice how in each case, the weight of the torso is supported by either the hands on the thigh or the hands on the floor.

My life is an expression of my mind, I surrender to my inner wisdom

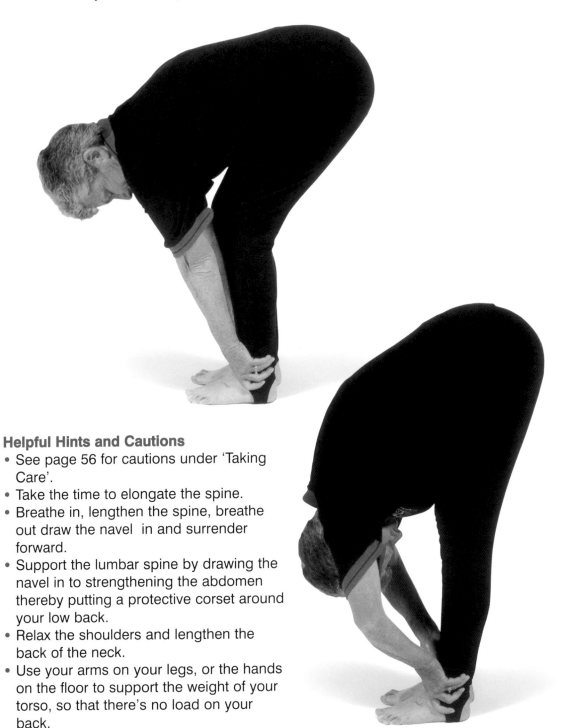

Helpful Hints and Cautions
- See page 56 for cautions under 'Taking Care'.
- Take the time to elongate the spine.
- Breathe in, lengthen the spine, breathe out draw the navel in and surrender forward.
- Support the lumbar spine by drawing the navel in to strengthening the abdomen thereby putting a protective corset around your low back.
- Relax the shoulders and lengthen the back of the neck.
- Use your arms on your legs, or the hands on the floor to support the weight of your torso, so that there's no load on your back.
- Bend your knees for safe practice if you have tight hamstrings.

Sitting and Twisting

The spine loves to be twisted. Twisting will stimulate body functions, improving posture, easing back pain, and relieving constipation. A flexible spine allows for a balanced upright posture allowing a free flow of information from the brain along the spine to every nook and cranny in your body by way of an amazing network of nerves.

Sitting Up, Not Down Sukhasana

Before beginning any sitting pose, take a moment to sit up, not down. When you sit on the floor or on a firm chair, you'll feel your sitting bones at the base of the pelvis. If you are sitting with a rounded spine, you're sitting on your spine as you compress the abdominal area. So, sit up , not down Ease back discomfort as you realign the spine and open the chest. Lengthen the front of the body, elongating the space between the pubis and the sternum, removing any frown lines across the belly! Belly smooth, shoulders relaxed down.

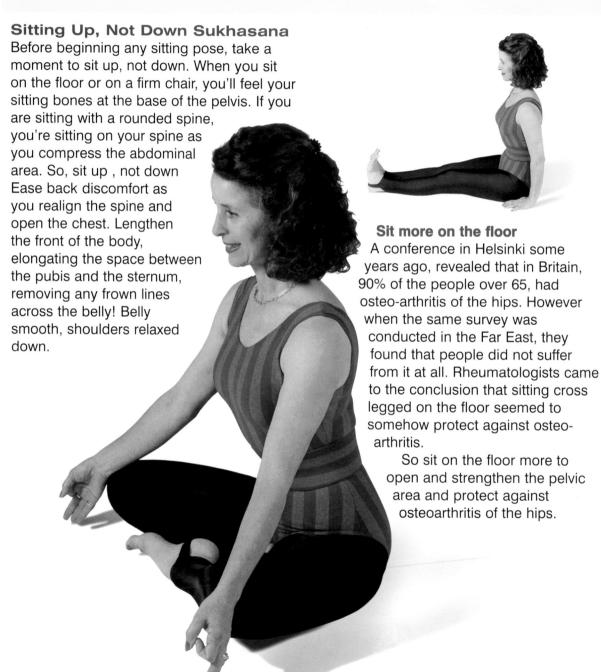

Sit more on the floor

A conference in Helsinki some years ago, revealed that in Britain, 90% of the people over 65, had osteo-arthritis of the hips. However when the same survey was conducted in the Far East, they found that people did not suffer from it at all. Rheumatologists came to the conclusion that sitting cross legged on the floor seemed to somehow protect against osteo-arthritis.

So sit on the floor more to open and strengthen the pelvic area and protect against osteoarthritis of the hips.

Don't forget that humanbeings are called 'homoerectus', not 'homocollapsus' or 'homoslumpus'!

Sitting and Twisting Matsyendrasana

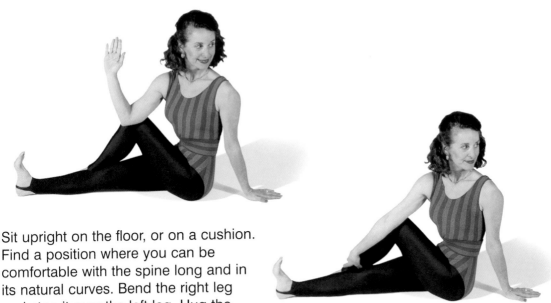

Sit upright on the floor, or on a cushion.
Find a position where you can be
comfortable with the spine long and in
its natural curves. Bend the right leg
and step it over the left leg. Hug the
knee towards you with the left arm.
Lengthen the spine upwards from the sitting bones right through the back of the neck up to
the crown of the head. When you're ready to twist, begin to spiral the spine from the base to
the crown, lengthening up on the inhalation and twisting a little further with the exhalation.
Draw the navel in from the thigh and allow your free
flowing breath to release any tightness along the spine.
Repeat on the other side.

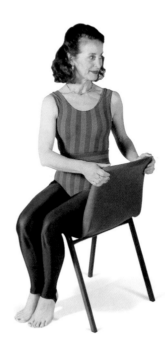

Chair Twist

Sit sideways on a chair, legs uncrossed. Spine straight
and rolling onto the front of the sitting bones. Elongate
the neck, tucking the chin in a little and twist so that you
can hold the back of the seat. Shoulders down, breathing
up the spine on the inhalation and twisting a little further
on the exhalation.

I focus on loving who I am, not hating who I am not

Practicing Together

Experience the joy of sharing and supporting, giving and receiving.
It is wonderful to feel the warmth and life rhythms of another. Experience a oneness.
In our world of 'them and us', give yourself a refreshing break and find someone, friend or partner and together experience a sense of union and harmony. The word yoga, means union, not separation. Practicing together will help you to overcome separateness and achieve union, as you deepen your relationship with your partner, friend or spouse.

Breathing Back to Back
Sit back to back allowing as much of the spine to touch as possible. Bring the buttocks close, and together begin to lengthen your spines all the way up to the back of the head. Now broaden the shoulders and feel the contact, the connection. Take a moment to tune into the rhythm of each other's breath. When you're ready to proceed further, link arms with each other so that the sensation of opening the chest is enhanced.

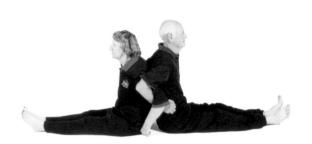

Row Row Row Your Boat
Begin by sitting face to face with the knees bent and the feet touching. Reach towards each other and hold hands for support. Take a few moments to let the spine lengthen with your breath and tune into each other. Relax the shoulders and smile.

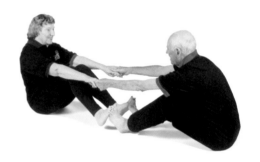

When you're ready, straighten one leg, pushing your feet together for strength. Now straighten the other leg, continuing to straighten the spine and lower the shoulders. Relax and enjoy letting the backs of your legs stretch a little further with each breath. Find the balance. Feel the stretch.

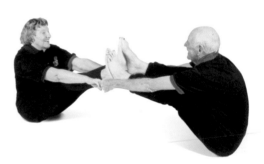

Now try rowing your boat to the destination of your best potential.

I experience the power of unconditional love, unconditional acceptance and unconditional approval.

I experience the power of unconditional self love, unconditional self acceptance and unconditional self approval.

Practicing Together

Try these supported backbend, forward bend and strength poses with your partner. Your combined rhythmic breathing will benefit both your postures. Trust your own natural intelligence to tell you whether these practices are suitable for you to try. Experience the joy of togetherness and the healing power of touch.

Backward and Forward Bend

One partner assumes swan pose with the body folded forward over the thighs and the arms lengthening in two straight lines beyond the head. Give your partner a chance to be comfortable, allowing the abdomen to settle on the thighs. Place your hands on either side of his spine and press down firmly with the weight of your body. Ask your partner if this is comfortable before you proceed. When you're ready, sit behind your partner and lean back over his low back before stretching over the swan posture. Let your hands touch. Breathing together, allow the swan pose to deepen, receiving your partner's stretch. Allow the backbend to open your heart. Stay in this position for several breaths allowing your emotions to merge into a peaceful awareness.

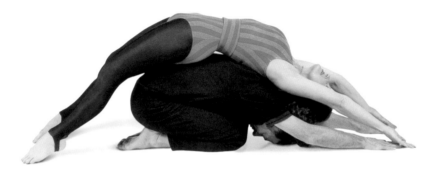

Back Bending Over Dog Pose

Let your partner assume dog pose, feeling steady, stable and strong, Press with the roots of the fingers to dynamically elongate the spine, flatten the upper back and lengthen the spine. Now gently lean back against your partner's upper back and roll onto your partner, back to back and hold the tops of his shoulders. Begin to experience your best back bend, feeling the loving support of your partner. Press the feet into the floor to allow your partner's spine to lengthen. Enrich the experience with your breath and your full attention. Back to back, united in strength.

Back to Back Shield of Strength
Begin in 'Shield Pose' (p61) Allow your partner
to build another shield behind you, mirror
image. Hold each other's ankle and reach up
to hold each other's hand. Take a moment to
gently allow your bodies to open and touch
all along the spine, the shoulders and the
back of the heads. Feeling strong together.

*I am ready. I am ready to receive. I am
ready to receive the healing that I need.
I am ready to receive. I am ready.*

*I am ready. I am ready to give. I am ready to
give the healing that you need. I am ready to
give. I am ready.*

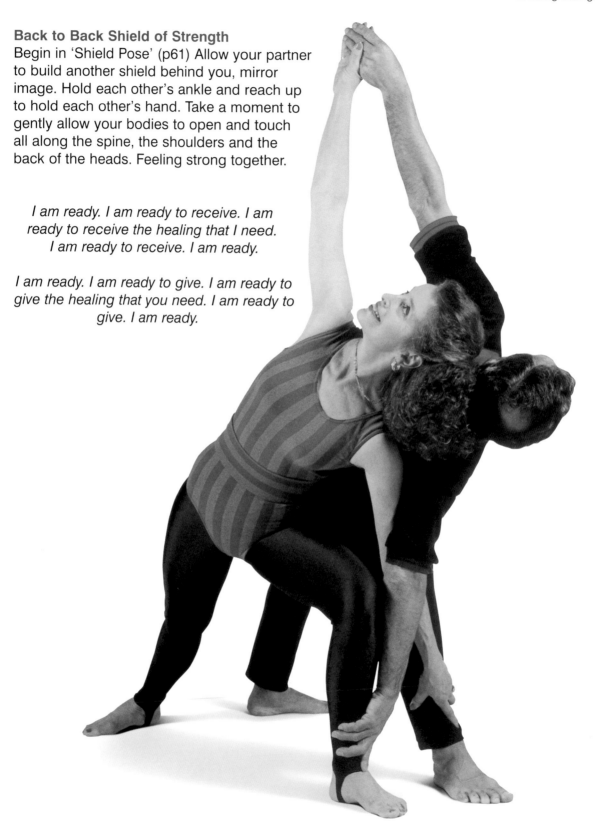

Side Stretching

Stretching to the side is something we rarely do in our every day activities. When we do, we benefit by opening the chest for better breathing and all along the sides of the spine to ease compression problems and relieve back pain. As you stretch to the side focus your awareness on elongating the short inner curve as well as the longer outer curve. Use your breath and abdominal tone to deepen the stretch.

Sitting Side Stretch For the Neck
Sit cross legged on the floor or upright on a chair if you prefer. Elongate the spine and roll onto the front edge of the sitting bones. Lengthen the back of the neck by drawing the chin in towards the sternum and allow the head to roll towards the right shoulder. Use the right hand across the top of the head as shown, to gentle deepen the stretch. If you need more stretch, lift the left arm alongside the left ear and allow the left side of the torso and neck to lengthen with your breath. Relax the right shoulder. Keeping the head where it is, allow the left arm to very slowly move to shoulder height, or even to the floor, so that you can experience a further stretch.

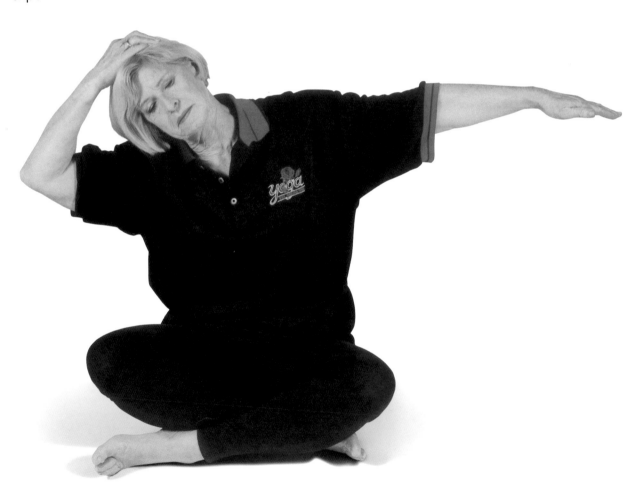

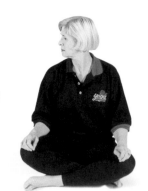

Release the stretch
Come back to centre, ears over the shoulders, face, eyes, throat soft, turn the head to one side nose towards shoulder. Draw some circles with the nose in both directions. Repeat both practices on the other side.

Standing Side Stretch
With the feet hip width apart, place your right hand on the right hip to support the torso. Stretch the left arm alongside the ear and begin to experience your best side stretch. Let your breath lure you deeper into the stretch and knowing when to stop. Repeat on the other side.

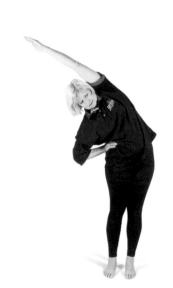

Growing Younger

Massaging your heart with your breath
The diaphragm is a muscular sheet at the base of the ribcage and separates the chest and abdominal cavities. The heart is the strongest muscle in your body yet only the size of your closed fist.

The heart rests on the diaphragm, snuggled between the lungs. Each deep conscious breath benefits the health of your heart.

Every breath you take, massages the heart. Take a few moments to experience the connection between your slow rhythmic breath and a slower pulse rate.

Kneeling Side Stretch

The Gate pose Parighasana

Begin in the kneeling position. Stretch the right leg out to the side and rest the right hand above the right knee. Stretch the left arm alongside the left ear and slowly begin to stretch over to the side without allowing the left shoulder to move out of alignment.

When your body invites you to stretch further, allow the right hand to move down the right leg a centimetre at a time. Work comfortably within your own range of motion.

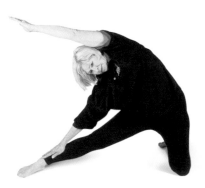

Release in child pose or swan pose before doing the other side.

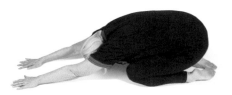

Swan pose

Growing Younger

Losing your mind

Contrary to popular belief, most elderly people do not suffer from Alzheimer's disease. Senility is a deterioration of mental abilities that can be related to other conditions which are largely preventable.

Many people are constantly dehydrated affecting the health of all the body's cells. So rediscover the delicious taste of nature's vintage and drink pure filtered water.

Vitamin deficiency and poor nutrition are other common causes of senility.

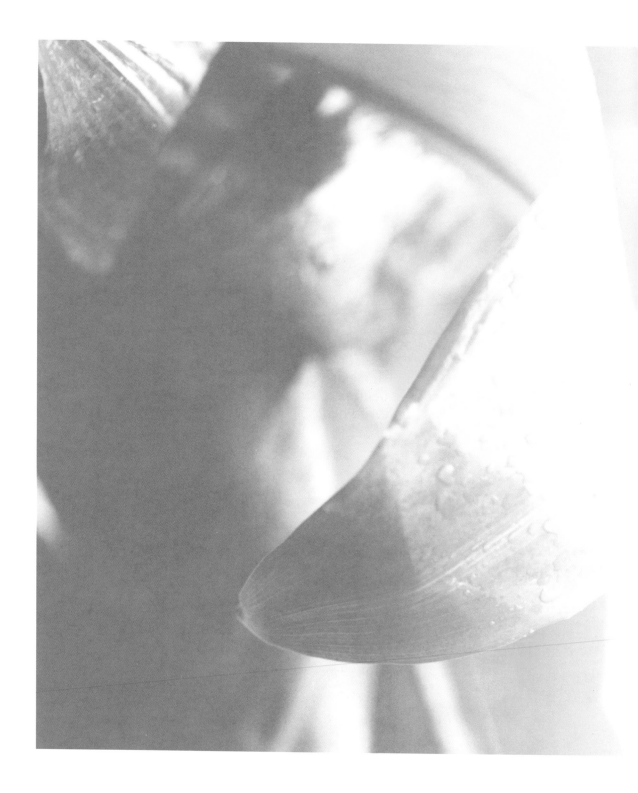

Growing a Younger Mind

Section3 Section3 Sectio

Meditation, Relaxation, Recipes, Gunas, Ganesha Your Body Is Your Vehicle

The Wise Woman's Precious Gem

One day while travelling through the mountains, the wise woman found a precious stone in a stream. She put it in her bag and continued on her journey. The next day she met a man who said that he was hungry, and asked to share her food. When she opened her bag, the man saw the precious stone and asked her to give it to him. To his surprise she did, without any hesitation at all.

The man left, rejoicing his good fortune. This precious gem would give him security for the rest of his life. However, on the next day he returned, looking for the woman. When he found her, he said, "I know how valuable this stone is, but I would like to give it back to you in the hope that you can give me something much more precious. Please share with me that which is within you, that empowered you to give me this precious stone in the first place".

If you want to know what your thoughts were like yesterday

Look at your body today.

If you want to know what your body will be like tomorrow

Look at your thoughts today.

(An old indian saying)

Meditation Dhyana

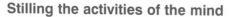

Stilling the activities of the mind

All our yoga practices prepare us for stillness in meditation.

A stiff, uncomfortable body and a stressed mind, are obstacles towards this end.

Yoga teaches that meditation is the stilling of the activities of the mind. We cannot ignore or stop our thoughts, but we can let them pass without attachment, judgment or evaluation. We can then slip beneath the busy activities of the mind and linger for a while in the vast spaciousness of our awareness; a place of stillness and bliss that is always there. Here we can tune into the natural intelligence of our own still calm centre and experience who we really are, ageless and timeless.

> ## Yoga teaches
> Still your mind. Still yourself and without doubt, you shall be united with the love that dwells in your heart.
> (Bhagavad Gita)

Preparing For Meditation

Find a comfortable place to sit where you won't be disturbed. Take the phone off the hook and look forward to this quiet time to be with yourself.

Take as long as you need to find a comfortable upright position so that the spine is erect allowing a free flow of awareness to pass between the brain, along the spine and to every part of your body. Allow the breath to settle. Experience the flow of relaxation and life force flowing up and down the spine in harmony with your relaxed, deepening breath. Waiting for the body to be ready for your meditation practice.

Meditation Practice

With the eyes gently closed, allow your focus to rest with the breath. Experience a soft warm golden light rising up the spine from the base of the spine to the crown of the head with each inhalation. With each exhalation, experience a flow of energy cascading from the crown over the shoulders caressing your body with relaxation, comfort and support.

Experience a strong inner support of strength at the very core of your being. Experience a deep sense of relaxation, acceptance and calm that envelopes your strength.

Experience the delicate balance between
strength and surrender
doing and being
getting and letting
receiving and giving

Experience harmony and balance. And this is yoga.

Enrich the experience of meditation with your breath and your complete attention.

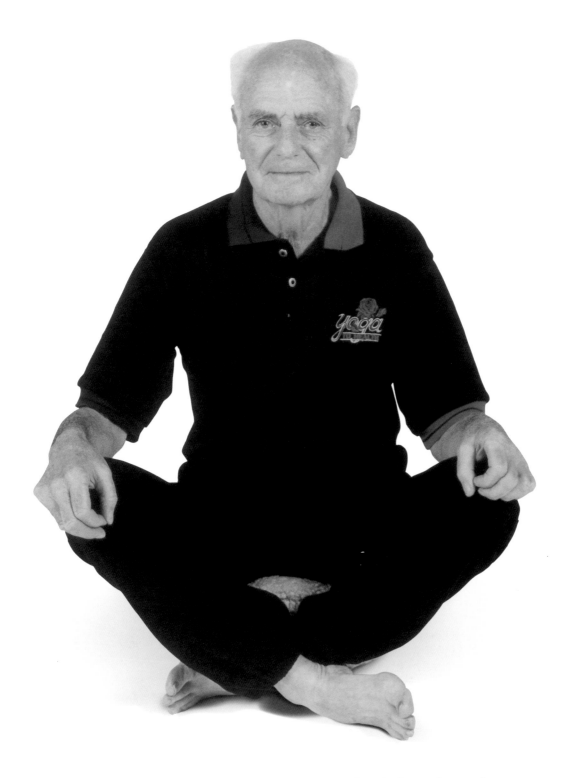

I am not by myself, I am with myself. I am not lonely, I am alone, all one.
I like the one I'm alone with.

Awareness Meditation Practice

Helping us to live in the present moment.
Yoga teaches that the only way to make rapid progress, is to progress slowly. Slowing down, allows for higher levels of awareness so that you'll know what's right for your unique self.

For this practice you'll need 2 almonds and a comfortable place to sit where you won't be disturbed.

Sit in a comfortable seated position either on the floor, on a cushion or on a chair. Take a moment to feel comfortable making sure that your spine is long and at ease. Experience your spine at rest in its natural curves. Very gently roll onto the front of your sitting bones and allow your spine to elongate a little more with each breath in, letting go any tension with each breath out. Experience your spine, simultaneously lengthening, straightening and relaxing.

Place the 2 almonds on your lap and sit quietly for a few moments until you feel ready to begin. Take one of the almonds and eat it until there is no residue left in the mouth. This is how you normally eat. Were you aware of the experience? Let's try eating the next almond with a greater focus on awareness, as you follow these instructions.

When you're ready, pick up the other almond and before placing it in the mouth, look at it, seeing its colour and texture. Smell it and see its size, shape and thickness. Where do you think it was grown? Draw strength from the miracle of nature that brought you this nutritious high calcium food. The sun, rain, tree, grower, picker transporter, all working in harmony. Now close your eyes and slowly place the almond on your tongue and experience its woody texture. Don't chew it yet! Let your tongue introduce the almond to your mouth and see how the mouth responds. Feel any saliva, your teeth, palate and cheek lining.

When you're ready, begin to slowly chew the almond for at least 30 bites before swallowing. Experience when the almond begins to taste like an almond and when it loses its flavour. Experience the intricate coordinating movements that are happening in your mouth. Enjoy the full experience. The experience of being fully aware and present in this moment. When you're ready to swallow, experience the process intimately, feeling the action in the throat, the descent of the pulp, following it to the stomach. Know that your body's natural intelligence will extract and keep what's needed and eliminate the rest. Now take a few moments to observe your breath with the same intimate awareness.

Tips for Everyday Breath Awareness

1. Take a short time to observe the quality of your breath every time you look at a watch or a clock. Is it smooth, even, quiet, long full, or is it shallow, jerky, anxious, tense?
2. Practice some full yoga breaths every time you stop at a traffic light or before breakfast or wherever! Breathing in lower, middle, upper. Breathing out, lower, middle, upper.
3. Observe the flow of your breath when you are holding a yoga posture that you find easy. Explore the effects of the breath.
4. Notice how breath is movement. Movements is life. Life is movement. Breath is life.

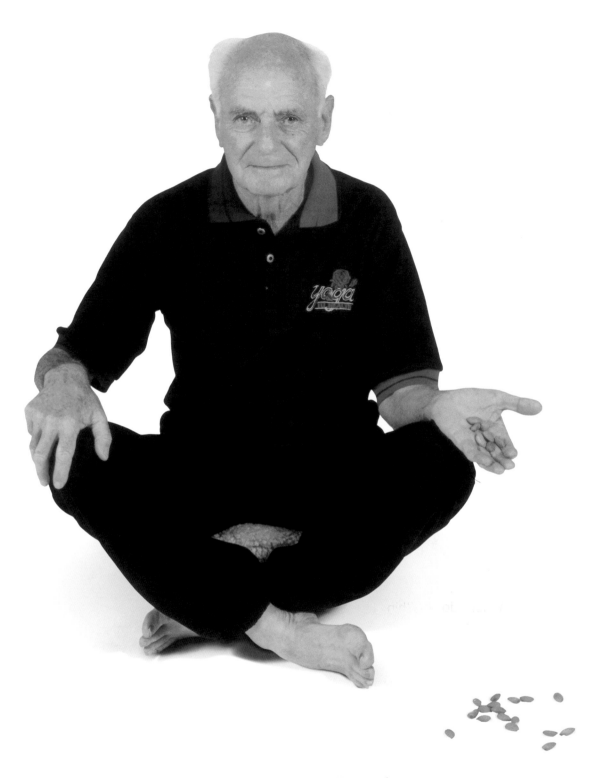

I am aware, I am awake. I linger in the stillness of my awareness.

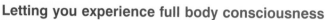

Relaxation

Letting you experience full body consciousness
Heightened awareness in relaxation is the practice of body consciousness. Allowing the mind to travel through the body to release excess tension so that there can be a free flow of energy through the body and the mind.

Yoga teaches that where the mind touches the body, the cells respond.
Let your mind touch your body. Let your body respond in healing and well being.

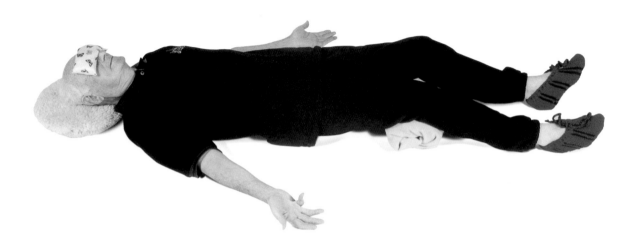

I am totally relaxed. I rest in the stillness of my inner calm. In stillness I heal.

Growing Younger

Breathing Slower, Living Longer
Yoga reminds us that when we are born we are allotted a certain number of breaths. When they are spent, we die.
So slow the breath, allowing it to gently deepen, soften and lengthen.

Preparing For Relaxation
Find a comfortable place for your relaxation practice. Take the phone off the hook so that you won't be disturbed. This is your special time. Lie down on the floor with the body's weight comfortably supported. You may need a small cushion under the head to relax and lengthen the back of the neck. You may need a rolled blanket behind the knees if the low back feels uncomfortable. You may like to use a small eye pillow and cover yourself with a light rug to stay warm. Spoil yourself with some yoga booties like the ones Fred is wearing.

Relaxation Pose Savasana
The relaxation pose is also called the dead man's pose. However it is more a posture of hibernation, than death.

The Relaxation Practice

You may like to record this text, reading it slowly or let someone read it to you.

- When you're ready, allow the legs to be a comfortable distance apart
- With the feet falling out to the sides.
- Allow the arms to roll away from the sides of the body
- With the palms turned upwards
- The fingers and thumbs lightly curled
- Let the navel sink down
- You may like to pinch the buttocks muscles together to relax the back
- Now relax the buttocks and the whole lumbar back.
- Elongate the back of the neck
- Drawing the chin towards the notch in the sternum
- Relax the whole head
- Relax the face
- With the eyes gently closed
- And the gaze turned down toward the stillness in the heart
- Relax all around the eyes
- Forehead, temples, relaxed
- Soften the face into a gentle smile
- Allow the jaw to be loose at the hinge
- With the lips lightly touching
- The teeth a little apart
- And the tongue relaxing in the floor of the mouth
- Whole face
- Whole body
- Comfortable
- Relaxed
- At ease.
- Allow your relaxed breath to gently deepen
- Making no effort, just letting it happen
- Allow waves of relaxation to radiate from your still calm centre into every nook and cranny of your body
- Seeking out any areas of discomfort
- Dissolving the discomfort and letting it go
- Allow the mind to find a resting place on the waves of your breath
- Whole body,
- Relaxed
- At ease
- Experience the support beneath your body
- And all that lies behind.
- Experience the space in front
- And all that is yet to come.
- Experience yourself in the present moment
- Between the past and the future
- Linger in the sensation of relaxation until you're ready to resume your daily activities.

Food for Life and Living

Improve the quality of your life by making more intelligent dietary choices. Look for calcium rich food. Look for organically grown produce in your area, or grow your own. Here you'll find 6 favourites that my students and I have enjoyed over the years.

I honour and respect this amazing machine called my body. I feed it only nourishing, fresh, healthy food. I am what I eat, think and do. I honour and respect my body.

Growing Younger

Senile Dementia

Although it is estimated that about 10% of elderly people show signs of senile dementia, clinical studies have shown that this can be slowed, stopped and even reversed by improved nutrition. It is common for elderly people to have a poor diet, lacking in nutrition.

Easy Fruit, Nut and Seed Slice

Contains no sugar and you won't believe how easy it is to make. Add any seeds of your choice. Dried fruit and nuts are rich in calcium and protein so you don't have to feel guilty having seconds!

3 cups mixed dried fruit with red and/or green cherries.
1 cup almonds and seeds of your choice (sesame, evening primrose, dry roast soy bean etc)
2 Tbsp flour and 3 eggs

Mix the flour into the fruit, nuts and seed mix to coat. Lightly beat the eggs to combine and stir into mixture. Spread into a greased lamington tin and press lightly. (I use an egg slice) Cook at about 180C for 30 minutes. Let cool and cut into pieces.

Hummous

Delicious, healthy, easy to make and rich in iron and calcium. It will store in the fridge for about a week. Serve with oven dried pitta bread and vegetable sticks. PS I use canned chickpeas occasionally.

1 cup chick peas soaked overnight
1/4 cup tahini (calcium rich sesame butter)
Clove of garlic
Juice of 1 lemon
Seasoning to taste (I use organic herb salt)

Place the drained peas in a saucepan, cover with cold water and boil for about 10 min. Simmer for up to 2 hours until soft. Strain, reserving the liquid. Place everything in the food processor or blender and blend with enough of the reserved liquid to make a creamy paste.

Wholemeal Almond Bread

Almonds are rich in calcium and protein. Keeps well in an airtight container, given half a chance!

1 cup SR wholemeal stone ground flour
150-200 gm almonds
4 egg whites
1/4 cup caster sugar

Beat the egg whites until firm and peaks form. Gradually add sugar and continue to beat until thick and glossy. Gently fold through the rest of the ingredients and spoon into the prepared greased loaf pan. Bake in a moderate oven for about 40 min at 180C. Turn out and wrap in clean tea towel overnight. Cut into very thin slices and place on a baking tray. Bake to dry at 140C for about 30 min.

Easy Spinach Quiche Slice

Delicious snack, entre or main vegetarian meal. Tastes wonderful either hot or cold.

1 packet frozen spinach, thawed and drained
1 cup grated or chopped mixed vegetables
1 large onion finely chopped
1 cup SR wholemeal flour
1/4 cup oil
5 eggs
1 cup low fat grated tasty cheese
1 chicken stock cube crumbled
Seasoning to taste (parsley, spring onions garlic organic herb salt, pepper etc)

Beat the eggs and combine all the ingredients mixing well. Pour into a loaf pan or greased spring form tin and bake in a moderate oven at 180C for 30-40 minutes or until browned.

Spinach Dip

Quick and easy to prepare, healthy and delicious to eat, economic and makes a large quantity.

1 packet frozen spinach
1 cup light sour cream or yogurt
1 cup light mayonnaise (try soy)
1 packet spring vegetable soup
Chopped spring onions and parsley to taste.

Thaw spinach and press out all the water. Mix in the rest of the ingredients. Refrigerate for an hour or so to thicken. Enjoy!

Date and Raisin Treat

No eggs. No sugar. Simply delicious healthy and fruity. Naturally sweetened and very more-ish!

1 cup chopped dates
3/4 cup raisins
3/4 cup orange juice
(or juice 2 oranges, grate the peel of one and drink the excess)
1 1/2cups SR wholemeal flour
1 tablespoon butter
3/4 cup finely minced almonds (I use food processor)
1 teaspoon vanilla essence
1/2 cup soy milk (or milk)

Put dates, orange juice and grated peel in a saucepan and heat through until the dates are soft. Remove from the heat and mash into a pulp. Stir through the butter and add the other ingredients. Stir well. Place in 2 buttered loaf pans and cook for 25 minutes at 180C. Cool, slice, enjoy, share, and store in an airtight container.

Growing Younger

Soy

Soy Beans are rich sources of natural oestrogen. Japanese women suffer less at menopause and have no word for 'hot flushes'. Best sources are whole organic soy beans not genetically altered. Look for them in tofu, temphe, soy drinks, soy mayonnaise and soy cheese. Find one you enjoy and add it to your daily diet.

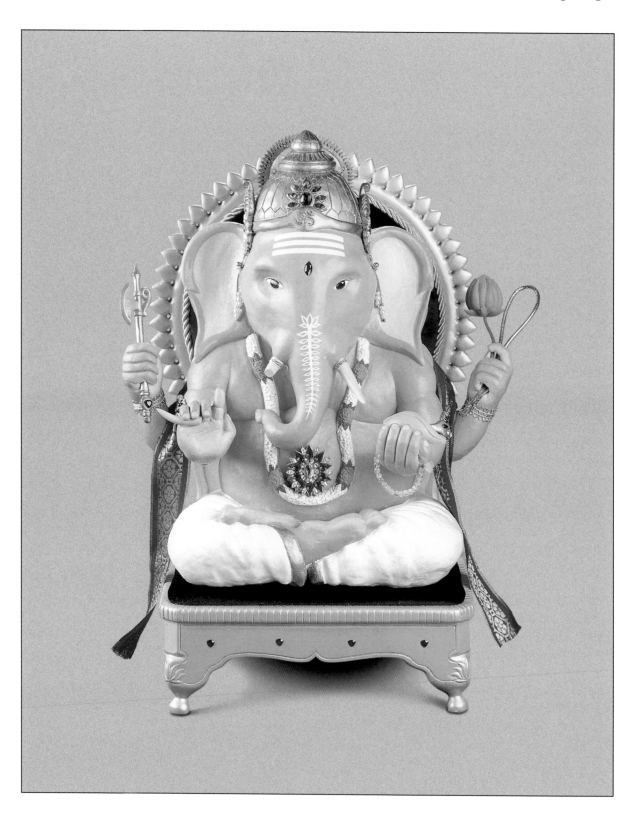

Ganesha

The remover of obstacles and your guide to fulfiling your dreams.

'My little brother and I spent many hours in our childhood sitting on grandpa's knee listening to wondrous tales of adventure. After he finished telling the story, we would always know the 'truth factor' by the last sentence in the story. 'And then an elephant came along and with his long trunk blew the story out!' He would then blow in our ears to make us laugh. He had such a charming way of making up tall tales that sounded so truthful. These fond memories of the relationship between elephants and mythology have always been perfectly natural with me!

Ganesha is a mythical Hindu elephant headed deity, very popular with the children. He is traditionally known as the remover of obstacles that we may encounter on life's journey. If however we perceive a situation as an obstacle, but Ganesha perceives it as an opportunity, the situation remains unchanged to become a learning experience for us. Ganesha will also place obstacles in the path of those who mean to do us harm.

Elephants have always been a seen as creatures of great wisdom, strength, support and intelligence and as such appear in many eastern ceremonies, celebrations and mythical tales. These strong and sensitive, noble and wise creatures are the earth's largest animals. Travellers who have encountered elephants on their journey often remark on the stillness that accompanies these gentle giants of the forest. They live in stillness in communities much like ours. They care for their young and their elderly and live about as long as we do.'

About Ganesha

- Ganesha is a loveable, fat, good natured deity with a healthy sense of humour to remind us that there are many situations in life that are not meant to be taken too seriously.

- He is the elephant headed, human bodied son of Parvati and Lord Siva and was born in the holy city of Varanasi on the River Ganges in North Eastern India.

- He has the head of an elephant with a broken tusk, a generous pot belly and uses a rat as his vehicle of transportation.

- Ganesha hears only the truth. Untruths are readily dispelled by a flap of the large ears.

- The long trunk breathes in the wisdom of the universe, connecting the inner and outer worlds.

- The tusks show strength, unity, resolve and oneness.

- The broken tusk not only symbolises the importance of letting the ego go, but is also said to have been used to write the epic story of the Mahabarata as dictated by sage Vyasa.

- The pot belly is abundant with the seeds of life.

- The rat vehicle demonstrates the overcoming of darkness and ignorance.

- With the head of an elephant and the body of a human, all earth's creatures are united.

The Gunas The 3 Forces of Nature

Have you noticed that one day you may feel enthusiastic and energetic, another day you may feel a bit flat and yet yesterday you felt so peaceful and calm. You wish you could feel like that all the time. Why can't you?

According to yoga philosophy, before energy is manifested in the world as we know it, all the natural forces were in perfect harmony and equilibrium. When manifested in the physical world, these forces can be individually defined. We can observe them and notice that at any one time, even though they are always all present, one of them will predominate. The gunas work at all levels of our being. Everything we do, feel and are, is in fact provoked by these 3 natural forces.

You'll find yourself smiling in amusement when you recognise these mischievous forces at work in your life.

You'll realise how natural change it is to change and evolve.

What Are These 3 Gunas?

1. Sattva Guna...being a human 'being'

Sattva is the natural force that maintains order. It is the innate impulse and inclination to evolve and grow. It is our impulse to be in harmony and to experience optimum health. It is our impulse to be human 'beings'.

2. Rajas Guna...being a human 'doing'

Rajas is the natural force to be active and energetic. It is the innate impulse to act. It is our natural desire to be busy and enthusiastic. It is our impulse to be human 'doings'.

3. Tamas Guna...being a human 'procrastinating'

Tamas is the natural force to do nothing. It is the innate impulse to remain the same. It is our natural desire to change nothing and to experience inertia. It is our impulse to be human 'procrastinatings'.

E-motion

Emotions are simply energies in motion. Emotions often cause disharmony in our life. We get caught up in them and aren't aware of their true nature. Emotions have motion.

They move. Just like the movement of the stars, tides, weather, seasons and day-night cycles, they are perfectly natural and in perfect order. The Gunas will help us to understand more about these natural forces of nature.

Which Guna is Dominant in You?

Knowing that these forces of nature are forever changing and that at any one time, any one of the 3 may predominate, it is interesting to see which guna predominates your personality most of the time.

A Sattvic Person

If you have a predominantly sattvic personality, you'll have the tendency to be satisfied, calm, centred and at peace with the world. You are likely to be a generous, caring person, truthful, gentle, humble and non violent. You will be looking to see how you may contribute to the welfare of your fellow human beings in selfless service. Sattvic people like to progress. Sattvic people will choose meditative practices such as meditation, t'ai chi and yoga as their preferred form of exercise.

A Rajasic Person

If you have a predominantly rajasic, personality, you'll feel more ambitious and competitive. You'll be driven to succeed, achieve and be better than others. You'll be more willful, energetic and impulsive. Your personality traits may include a tendency to be affectionate, envious, deceitful, materialistic and proud. Rajasic people like to be active, their attention scattered and their desires insatiable. Rajasic people will choose dynamic and stimulating, competitive forms of exercise.

A Tamasic Person

If you have a predominantly tamasic personality, you'll have the tendency to feel depressed, dull, bored and flat. You'll be lacking energy and drive. You'll display tendencies towards being conceited, ignorant, cruel, offensive and boring. Tamasic persons like to restrain. They have the tendency to endlessly postpone and live a self centred life style. Tamasic people aren't interested in any form of exercise.

Yoga teaches

Our body is composed of atoms and molecules. These are arranged as cells, tissues organs and systems to form our human organism by an animating life force. Yoga teaches that all life comes from nature, from a central force called PRAKRITI. When we die, PURUSHA, the soul is released. The life force that flows through our being is called PRANA. Prana is the gross manifestation of purusha.

We All Have All Three

We can all relate to all three tendencies at one time or another. Yoga practices help you to be aware of these tendencies and to help you to make intelligent choices towards the kind of person you want to be.

Yoga teaches

All our actions, feelings and choices are provoked by the gunas.
Which of the guna predominates in you right now?.

Sattva

It's time to turn off the TV. I'd like to meditate for 10 minutes before I go to bed.

Tamas

Stay up and watch the late night movie. I don't want to move from here.

Rajas

Hurry up and make up your mind!

	Sattva	Rajas	Tamas
Food	Nourishing, pure, natural foods, fruit, vegetables, nuts, juices, milk, honey, cereals, wholemeal bread, water, herbal teas	Over-stimulating, hot, spicy, salty, fish, eggs, chocolate, caffeine.	Tasteless, overcooked, overripe, fermented foods, meat, alcoholic beverages
Health	Ease	Disease	Sluggishness
You	Peaceful, serene	Impulsive, willful	Lacking enthusiasm, ignorant
Your breath	Space between the breaths	Inhale	Exhale
The weather	Calm, sunny, warm and beautiful	Stormy, windy, blowing, changing	Humid, overcast, foggy
Emotions	Calm, serene, content, centred	Angry, excited, afraid, ambitious	Depressed, sickly, sad
Colours	White, gold, pink, pastels, blue, mauve	Red, orange, yellow, bright, bold, brilliant	Brown, black, dark, grays, faded.
Feelings	Joy, contentment	Pleasure, jealousy	Pain, ignorance
Seasons	Spring, autumn	Summer	Winter
Tides	Changing tides	Ebb	Flow
Temperature	Mild, just right	Hot	Cold

Looking at a Garden

The world we perceive consists of created matter viewed in combination of how we interpret that matter through the use of our senses. This interpretation is very much dependent on which guna predominates at the time.

Below is an example of how three different people can view a garden according to which natural guna force is most active at the time. The garden is the same. The weather and the plants are the same. Yet they may be viewed and enjoyed very differently.

A Sattvic Person

What a glorious day. The lighting this morning is magnificent. There are quite a few butterflies around. I can see them landing softly on the daisies. It looks as if the roses will soon be in full bloom. I can see some birds preparing a nest. I think I'll spend a few moments in silent appreciation of this lovely place.

I am at peace.

A Rajasic Person

The weeds have grown quickly. We have friends visiting this afternoon, I'll quickly do some weeding. I'll remove the rubbish and prune the roses. If I hurry, I can do that now before lunch.

I'd better not waste any time.

A Tamasic Person

All gardens look the same to me. It is just another garden. I don't see what all the fuss is about. That lazy chair looks good. I think I'll go over there and have a little snooze. This is a boring day.

I am feeling tired.

As I seek growth, I find growth in everything I experience.

Your Body Is Your Vehicle

Your body is the mobile home that you live in. It is the precious vehicle that takes you from place to place, safely and on the whole, faithfully. Compared to our car or house however, we tend to neglect our own body and often wait for it to break down before we think about maintenance. Yoga practices give us the right tools to maintain our vehicle's optimum performance.

Just like a car, it involves 10 main aspects for sound performance and appearance.

1. A Bright Shiny Body
By remaining active and flexible, the whole body is nourished, the skin radiant and your eyes bright and alive.

2. A Clean Interior
Breathing and posture practices stimulates the elimination, digestion and lymphatic systems to function more efficiently.

3. A Lubrication System
Yoga postures move systematically, to stimulate, move and strengthen all the joints in the body. These well thought out postures, encourage the joints to remain well lubricated with the body's natural fluids.

4. A Well Charged Battery
Deep, rhythmic breathing allows you to recharge your body's energy stores. Experience your solar plexus as your energy storage centre. Every deep, full, complete breath tops you up with new reserves of energy and vitality.

5. A Cooling System
Relaxation practices allow your body and mind to cool down as they release accumulated tension. Relaxation is your whole being's natural cooling system.

6. Clean Appropriate Fuel
A sensible, wholesome, natural, fresh, balanced diet, is the preferred diet for efficient functioning of your body's organs and systems. Just as you wouldn't expect your car to run smoothly on anything other than the correct fuel, your body also needs the correct fuel for your unique vehicle.

7. A Sound Suspension
Awareness and posture practices will create optimal alignment and balance for ease of movement so that your vehicle is able to take you comfortably wherever you want to go.

8. A Navigator
Self study, meditation, introspection and self exploration, will help you to be more aware of the best route to take on your journey through life.

9. A Purpose
All the practices of yoga allow you the opportunity to turn within and experience yourself in stillness. Within this stillness you'll be able to tune into your body's natural intelligence and discover your unique purpose in life.

10. A Trained, Licensed Driver
Still your mind. Go within. Know yourself. Become the responsible driver to safely guide your vehicle in the direction of your choice.

I have the **strength**

To hold my **stillness** within

And keep it **safe** from outside hurts

And my own **thoughts**.

To hold this **stillness** in my heart

And in this **effort** I will not cease

And in this way, I keep my **peace**.

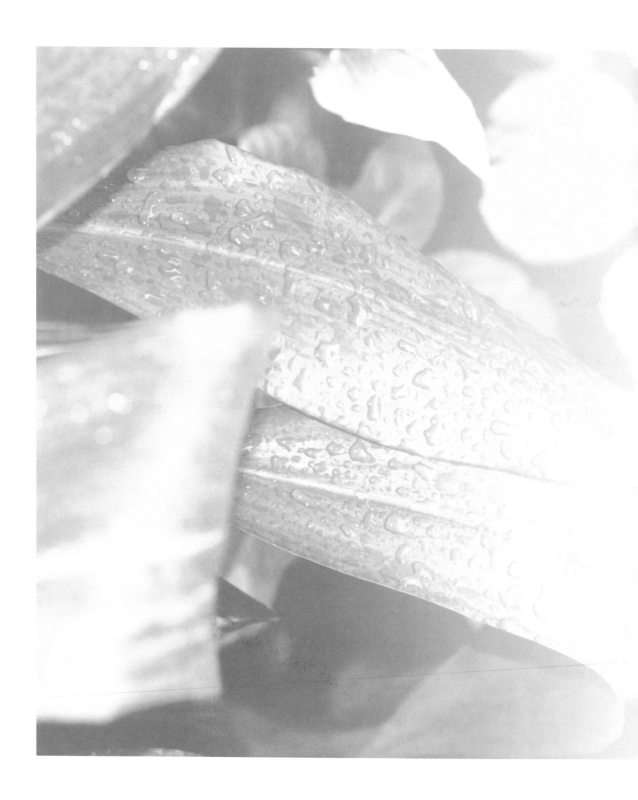

Keeping You Young

Practice Routines

In this section you will find practice routines to keep you young. The routines incorporate many of the poses that have been outlined earlier. Practicing each day constitutes a daily commitment to be with yourself, to value yourself, to focus in the present moment and to tune into your unique needs at this time. It takes only a short time and your body will thank you for it in terms of greater vitality and an enhanced feeling of well being.

During your daily yoga practice routine, you'll have the opportunity to turn within and experience yourself at all levels of being. You'll find that at the beginning you may have to drag your body to your daily practice routine, but in time your body will drag you, because it makes you feel so good.

What you need
1. A resolve to take charge of your own well being
2. A quiet, uncluttered place where you won't be disturbed
3. An empty stomach (about 2 hours)
4. You may also like to use a strap, a blanket or rug, a small pillow and a bolster.

Do the Dog
A whole practice routine in one pose

How old do you feel?
Aging is the gradual loss of mental and physical ability. The body stiffens, the breath becomes shallow and vitality is lost. This will make you feel old. Your body wants to be well. It wants to breathe. It knows how to heal and renew itself. All you have to do is allow it to happen. In this section, you'll have the opportunity to find a practice routine to suit your unique needs. Find a practice that you enjoy, so that you will want to do yoga everyday.

With every breath I take, I breathe into my body and my mind, the breath of unconditional love. The breath of unconditional self love, self acceptance and self approval.

Practice Routine 1

Asthma and Arthritis (allow about 5 minutes)
My body, my mind and my breath are bathed in stillness and calm.

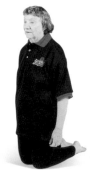

1. Begin by kneeling with the feet and knees as wide as the hips. Support the lumbar region by gently firming the buttocks muscles and drawing the navel in towards the spine. Experience the strength supporting the low back. You may feel more comfortable with a cushion under the knees.

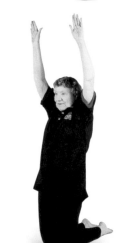

2. When you're ready to inhale, allow the back of the neck to lengthen and the arms the effortlessly drift up beyond the head, keeping the arms shoulder width apart. Reach and lengthen, waiting for the end of the inhalation.

3. When you're ready to exhale, spread the arms wide like wings and begin to move forward by first of all sitting back towards the heels. Ease the body forward, allowing the tummy to rest on the thighs, the shoulders to move down away from the ears, with the arms lengthening towards the feet, fingers resting by the toes. Allow the forehead to rest on the floor, neck long and comfortable. If you have blood pressure problems see the modified child pose on page 40.

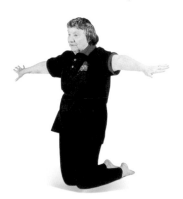

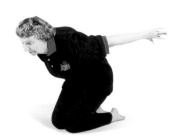

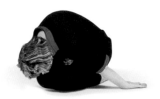

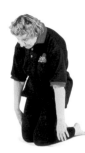

4. When you're ready to breathe in, draw the navel in, tuck the chin in and uncurl one vertebra at a time bringing the head up last. You may like to rest in the thunderbolt position for several breaths before repeating the routine 5 more times.

Stillness and Calm

See the mind as a deep pond. At the bottom of the pond it is still and calm. Here lies the true Self.

Know that we can only see the bottom when the pond is clear and still. Only then can we see its full depth. If the mind pond is muddy and agitated, the bottom of the pond will remain hidden from view. Yoga practices of stretching, relaxing and breathing help to clear and calm the mind pond any time we choose so that we can experience our true self.

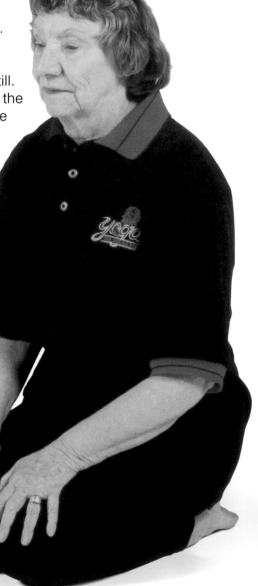

Practice Routine 2

Spine Savers for Back Pain (allow about 20 minutes)

I am completely satisfied with my body, my mind, my life, myself. I am completely satisfied.

1. Semi-supine position

The semi-supine position is the best resting position for the back. Position the knees and the feet as wide as the hips. Wait for your body to soften into the floor. Feel the low back at ease against the floor.

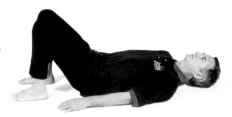

2. Full body stretch

Stretching the arms beyond the head, rotating the ankles, breathing deeply.

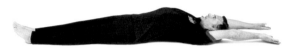

3. Spine stretch

With the finger over or under the knees, draw the nose towards the knees, neck long, shoulders down elbows wide

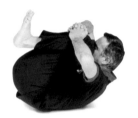

4. Pelvic tilt

Tilt the pelvis in harmony with your breath, exhaling letting the navel sink down heavily, inhaling letting the low back arch away from the floor. Experience the release of tension all around the lumbar area.

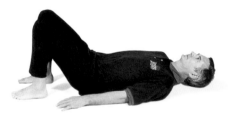 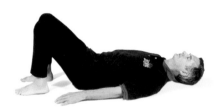

Growing Younger

Calcium

For calcium to be absorbed most efficiently, it needs a low acid environment and the presence of vitamin D. So enjoy our abundant sunshine and protect the calcium in your body by including in your diet, a daily drink of diluted apple cider vinegar, honey, lemon juice and calcium and/or sodium ascorbate, a powerful vitamin C antioxidant.

Did you know that celery contains special anti arthritic minerals? You'll love it juiced with carrots, apple and pineapple!

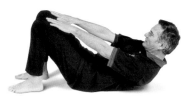

5. Abdominal strength

Rest the hands on the thighs. Lengthen the back of the neck and allow the low back to rest comfortably on the floor, Feet and knees still hip width apart. On the exhalation, contract the lower abdomen, pressing the low back into the floor. Now lift the head and shoulders a little and experience the abdominal wall strengthening. Repeat 10 times, knowing that sit-ups a day will keep the back doctor away.

6.hamstrings

Put a strap around the sole of the right foot and allow the leg to straighten as much as it comfortably can. Experience the stretch behind the back of the thigh and behind the knee. Let each exhalation gently lead you to your best stretch sensation. Simply breathe and wait for your hamstrings to find their best stretch. Enjoy the sweet discomfort of release. Repeat with the left leg.

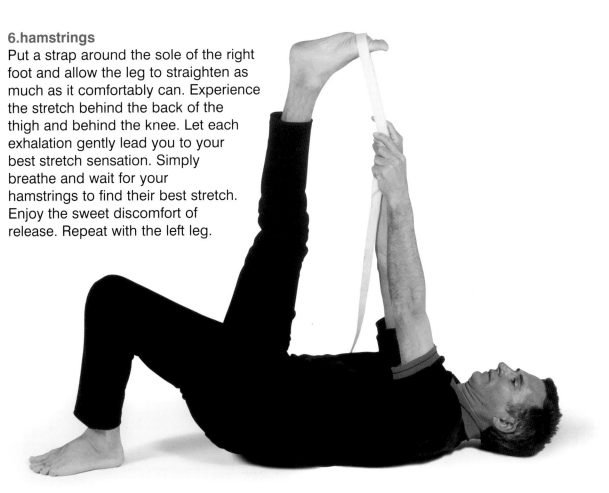

7. Back massage

Hug the knees to the chest and roll from side to side, massaging the muscles along the spine from the buttocks to the shoulders

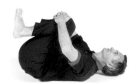

8. Supine twist

Keeping the feet and ankles together, roll the knees to the right as you roll the head to the left. Make sure that the back of the neck is long, the arms at shoulder height, palms down. Smile. To stretch further, rest the right hand on the knees, breathing rhythmically and easily, allowing the spine to spiral and loosen in its own good time. Do other side.

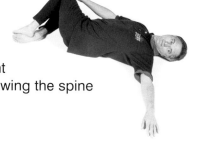

9. Cat stretch

Roll to the right and push yourself onto all fours. Position the hands under the shoulders and the knees under the hips. Lengthen, straighten and flatten the spine. Exhaling, draw the navel in and arch the spine towards the ceiling, tucking the tail under. Inhaling, lift the tail, lower the waist, lift the head looking up. Do 6 more rounds in harmony with your breath.

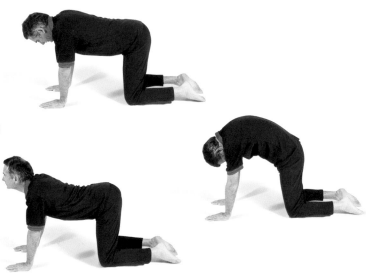

10. Dog pose

Allow your strong arms and legs to lengthen, strengthen and elongate the spine dynamically. See p62-63

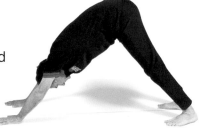

11. Frog pose

Spread the knees wide and allow the big toes to touch. Fold forward with the arms lengthening beyond the head in 2 straight lines releasing shoulder tension and allowing you to breathe deeply and rhythmically.

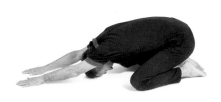

12. Sit back on the heels
Close the eyes and take a moment to experience the benefits of the practice.

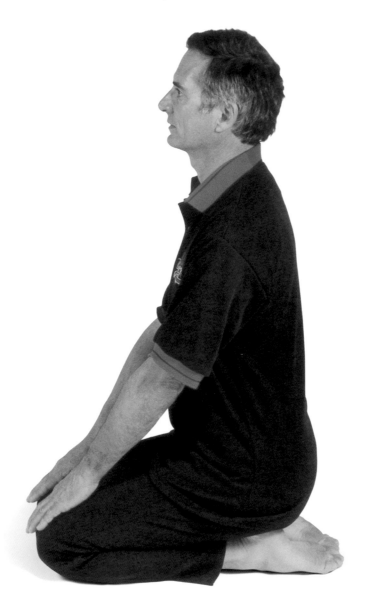

Growing Younger

Loosen Up

A cat is a picture of looseness and fluidity. See how smoothly it moves and how that relates to how relaxed it is. Just pick it up and let it droop over your hand.

Know that tension held in the body, causes the muscles to contract. We then have stiffness in the joints. Circulation is impeded and sooner or later disease sets in the form of arthritis, inflammation and joint discomfort. So emulate your cat with its smooth. fluid movement, relaxed limbs, alert yet relaxed, its joints loose,limp and limber.

Practice Routine 3

Strength and Flexibility (allow about 10 minutes)
I have the power within me to create for myself a life of peace, fulfilment and joy.

1. Mountain pose
Beginning your practice in mountain pose and tune into your body's natural strength and alignment. Breathing deeply into the solar plexus, whilst simultaneously grounding and growing from your deep calm centre of strength.

2. Warrior pose
Spread the feet wide apart, turning the right foot out and the left foot in and sinking down into the strength of warrior pose. Repeat on the other side.

3. The Half Triangle pose
Rest the right elbow on the knee and wrap the left arm around the waist. Take a moment to align the spine, strengthen the legs and open the body. Breathe spaciousness into the joints with each inhalation and let go deeper into the pose with each exhalation.

4. The Triangle pose, or Shield pose
If your body asks for a further stretch, deepen the pose into the shield pose with the back of the hand against the instep and the fingertips a millimetre off the floor. Breathe and smile. Repeat 2-4 on the other side.

Growing Younger

Move it or lose it
Everyone over the age of 25 begins to show signs of spinal degeneration. However, by moving your joints without pain, will improve not only the supply of nutrients to the joints but also help to strengthen the bones.
So move it, or you'll lose it.

---

5. Dog pose
Release the spine in dog pose, using the arms and legs strongly to lengthen and straighten the spine while strengthening the spine and joints of the whole body.

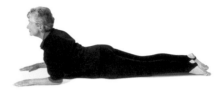

6. Sphinx pose
Drop the knees to the floor, lying down on the front of the body. Prop yourself up onto the forearms, elbows under the shoulders and allow the spine to soften into sphinx pose.

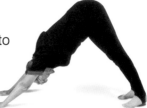

7. Child pose
Recover in child pose, letting the whole body soften as you tune into the rhythmic ebbing and flowing of the breath.
Now repeat 1-7 on the other side.

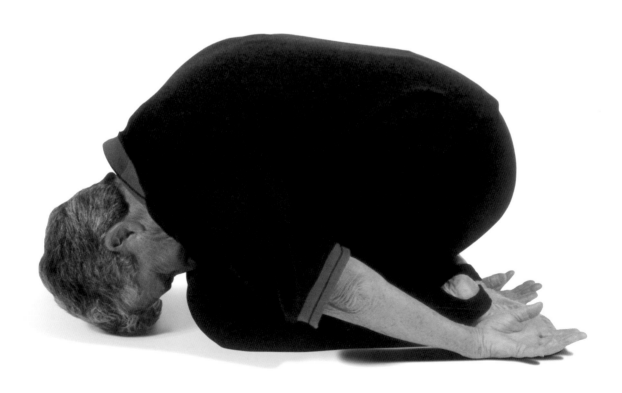

Relax and Rejuvenate (allow about 15 minutes)
In stillness I heal my body, my mind and my emotions. In stillness I heal.

1. Legs Up The Wall
Rest the legs up the wall with the buttocks as close to the wall as possible. Lengthen the back of the neck, relax the shoulders, soften the face, eyes and throat.

2. Preparing For Shoulder Stand
Bend the knees and place the feet hip width apart on the wall. Experience a gentle stretch in the lumbar back. Breathe relaxation energy through your entire being.

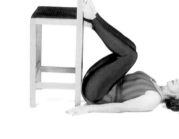

3. Pushing The Wall Away
Press the feet into the wall, lifting the buttocks off the floor and inhaling. Lower the buttock onto the floor as you exhale. (See 'Taking Care' caution on p56)

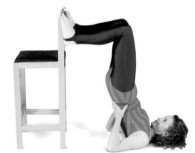

4. Supported Half Shoulder Stand
You may be able to lift a little higher on your next inhalation, squeeze the muscles along the pelvic floor and experience this inversion for the abdominal viscera and an elongation for the neck.

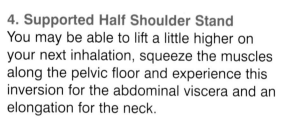

5. Hug Yourself
Hug the knees to the chest and experience a gentle stretch in the low back, hamstring and buttocks.

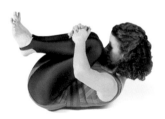

Growing Younger

Liberating the feet

In many Asian countries such as India and Japan, people wear shoes only when necessary. The feet are then released from constriction and discomfort and feel so much better. The house stays cleaner and quieter, as you experience the richness beneath your feet of all the textures that you didn't know existed. Take off your shoes and experience the prickly grass, the soft sand, the smooth carpet, the textured tiles. Your feet will love you forever!

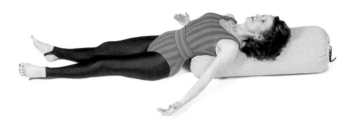

6. Opening The Chest

Once you experience the chest opening benefits of this pose, you'll want to practice it every day. Improved deep breathing and better posture will be your reward. Use rolled blankets or a bolster long enough to comfortably support the whole torso and head.
Make sure the neck is long. You may need a small cushion under the head. To open the hips, practice this pose with a strap around the feet. Simply breathe and relax, allowing your body to receive the stretch.

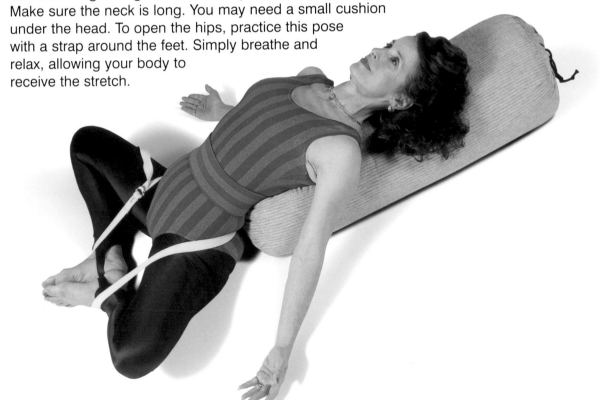

The Seven Way Stretch (allow about 5 minutes)
This easy flowing standing sequence will help you to stretch the spine through its full range of motion.

   It is an excellent preparation before you do your standing poses.
You may even like to do this sequence on its own to simply enliven your spine and uplift your spirits.

1. Stretching Up
Interlace the fingers. Breathe in turning the palms towards the ceiling. Chin in, shoulders down, inner arms hugging the ears, tailbone lengthening towards the floor. Lengthen the spine a little more with each inhalation. Relax the shoulders and lengthen the tailbone a little more with each exhalation. Experience the spine lengthening.

I reach, I grow, I am grounded.

2. Stretching To One Side
With the fingers still interlaced above the head and the palms still turned upwards towards the ceiling, inhale, and reach higher. Exhale, relax the shoulders down, neck long, navel drawn in, push the rib cage to the left as you stretch to the right. Experience the stretch all the way from the left heel to the fingers, opening the whole left side of the body. Experience the rib cage opening.

I am open to all the possibilities of life.

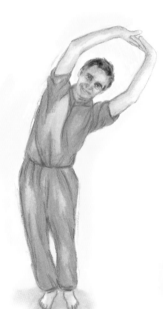

3. Stretching To The Other Side
Inhale, coming back to centre. Exhale, lower shoulders down and with the, neck long and navel drawn in, push the rib cage over to the left side. Experience the stretch all the way from the right heel to the fingers, opening the whole right side of the body. Experience the rib cage opening on this side.

As I open my body, I open my mind.

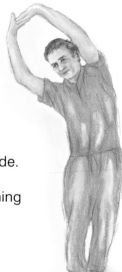

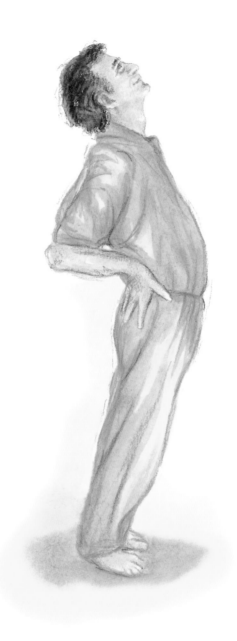

4. Stretching The Spine Backwards

Place the hands on the buttocks, lengthening the low back by pushing the buttocks down and the hips forward. Soften the knees. Allow the chest to open with the inhalation as you allow the spine to extend a little further backwards with the exhalation. Experience the front of the spine stretching and lengthening.

I receive. I am receptive to the abundance of the universe.

5. Stretching The Spine Forwards

Bend the knees and rest the hands on the thighs. Take a moment to elongate the spine with your in-breath. Now place the abdomen on the thighs and allow the body to cascade forward. Continue to look up if you have blood pressure problems. If you're comfortable, hold the ankles and gently allow the legs to straighten just a little at a time., with the abdomen still resting on the thighs, supporting the lumbar back. Experience the whole back of the body stretching.

I surrender.

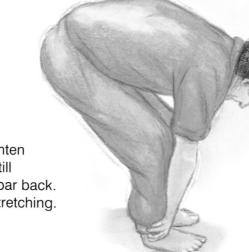

6. Twisting To One Side

With the arms at shoulder height, place the left hand on the right shoulder and gently push yourself to the right as you allow the spine to twist. Follow the movement with your eyes. Stop and take another breath in and see if you can push yourself around a little further.

I am aware. I am awake.

7. Twisting To The Other Side

When you're ready, come back to centre and place the right hand on the left shoulder and gently push yourself to the left as you allow the spine to twist. Follow the movement with your eyes. Stop and take another breath in and see if you can push yourself around a little further.

I am ready. I am ready to receive the healing that I need.

Now that you've finished the 7-Way stretch, shrug the shoulders up around the ears and rest the back of the head on the little cushion that you've made. When you're ready to release, gather up any shoulder tension that you can find, and release it as you lower the shoulders, relaxing them away from the ears. Experience the tension flowing down the arms into the fingers and dripping onto the floor.

Bouncing Back To Health

(Allow about 5 minutes)
It's fun, it's simple and for reasons not fully understood, it really works!
Get yourself a 'rebounder' and bounce back to health and strength. Invest in a good quality one and allow it to help you to strengthen your muscles and bones without strain or tension. Take it gently at first to feel your centre and your balance. Now relax, breathe evenly and rhythmically and enjoy the experience, letting your body unfold when it's ready.

Listen to your own natural intelligence to tell you whether this practice is right for you. When's the last time you did something like this?

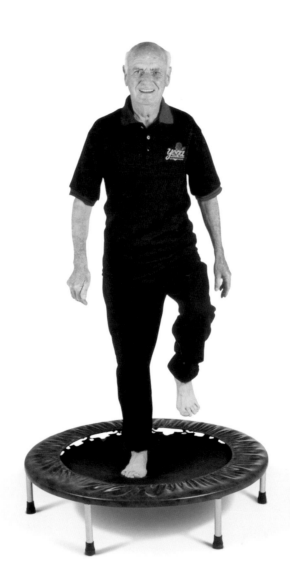

'Hey, this feels wonderful! I feel like a kid again.' said Fred when he first tried the rebounder.

My Own Daily Practice Routine

You are now ready to build your own unique balanced practice routine. Simply fill in the blanks and it's there.

Follow the Kiss principle... Keeping It So Simple

Affirmation

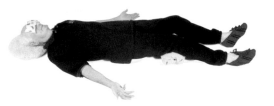

1. Relaxation Pose p96
To release tension from the body and mind

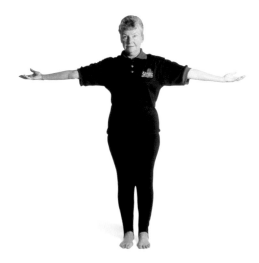

4. Moving Breath Meditation p29

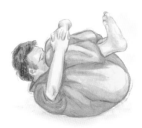

2. Warming Up p53
Choose 3 warm up poses

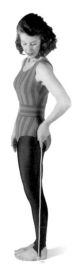

3. Mountain Pose p52 - To align the spine.

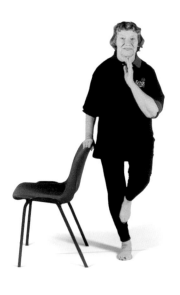

5. Balance p76-77
Choose 1 standing balance pose

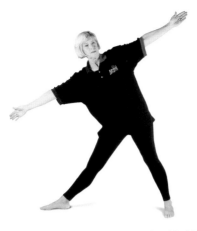

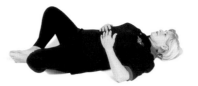

10. Breathe p31, 35, 37
Choose 1 breathing practice

6. Standing Poses p52, 60, 67, 81, 120
Choose 2 standing poses

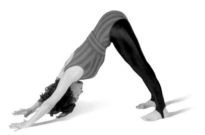

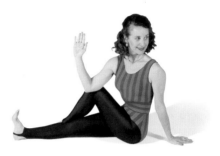

11. Twist p83
Choose 1 twist pose

7. Dog Pose p62

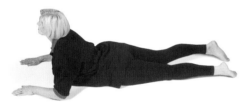

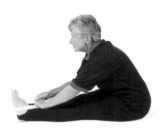

12. Sitting Forward Bend p80
Choose 1 forward bend pose

8. Sphinx Pose p78

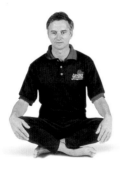

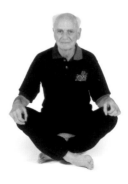

13. Relaxation, Meditation P92-96
Choose 1 or 2 practices

9. Sit and Stretch p82. Choose one sitting pose

125

You'll enjoy the 'Sun Salute' series of postures more and more with practice. You're body will be bursting for more in no time! Here Fred and I show you the full version and a modified version that suits you best. Repeat the sequence with the left foot lunge. This is one complete round. Do several more rounds if your body asks for more.

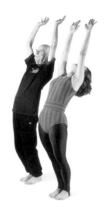

Sunburst
inhaling, tailbone lengthening towards the heels.

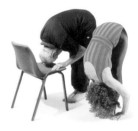

Forward Bend
exhaling

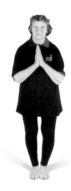

Namaste
exhaling with the palms of the hands together at the centre of the chest.

Salute To The Sun

Salute to the sun is an ideal way to begin your practice. It can be used as a warm up routine or you could slow it down and use it as a flowing daily practice. In class we often perform it to various versions of Pachelbel's Canon and may add a posture like triangle pose to make it an even more balanced practice.

You'll notice that each posture counterposes the one before and alternates between expanding and contracting the chest and between bending the spine backwards and forwards. If you want a dynamic

Begin Here

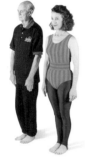

Mountain Pose
feeling centred, grounded and ready.

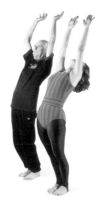

Sunburst
inhaling, opening the front of the body. Shoulders down.

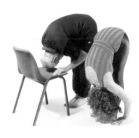

Forward Bend
exhaling

Growing Younger

I'm OK

For a whole week, make a promise to yourself that at least four times everyday, you'll pass by a mirror, stop and look at yourself directly in the eyes, smile and say, 'I'm OK!'

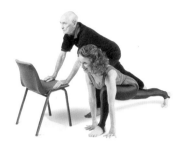

Right Foot Back Lunge
inhaling, knee directly over the ankle

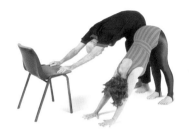

Dog Pose
exhaling

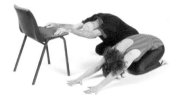

Swan Pose
Sitting back on the heels having a rest.
Suspending the breath.

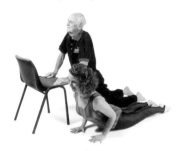

Cobra
inhaling, shoulders down, neck long, navel
drawn in, big toes pressing into the floor.

practice follow the breathing suggestions. If you want to slow it right down, simply allow the breath to flow freely at all times.

Have fun. Challenge yourself by gradually building the number of rounds to 10.

Experience the balance of your grounding and growing energies. Experience the balance between opening and closing: giving and receiving. Experience the connection between what the American Indians call mother earth and father sky.

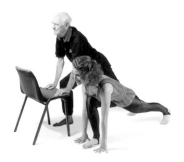

Right Foot Forward Lunge
inhaling, knee directly over the ankle.

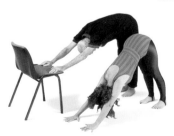

Dog Pose
exhaling

Further Reading

There are so many excellent publications on the market. Here are some suggestions. Look for some yourself in Health Food stores, Metaphysical bookshops, book stores and second hand book shops.

Look under yoga, health, and new age for inspiration.

Ageless Body, Timeless Mind
Deepak Chopra . . . .*Random House 1993*

Quantum Healing
Deepak Chopra . . . .*Bantum 1990*

You'll See it When You Believe It
Wayne Dyer . . . .*Bookman Press 1989*

Yoga, the Spirit and Practice of Moving into Stillness
Erich Schiffman . . . .*Pocket Books 1996*

The New Yoga for People over 50
Suza Francina . . . .*Health Communications Inc 1997*

The Breathing Book
Donna Farhi . . . .*Simon and Schuster 1997*

Light on Yoga
BKS Iyengar . . . .*The Aquarian Press 1976*

The Upanishads
Juan Mascaro . . . .*Penguin 1965*

The Bhagavad Gita
many versions

The Book of Yoga
Sivananda Yoga Centre Book Club Associates 1985

Awakening the Spine
Vanda Scaravelli . . . .*Harper Collins 1991*

Yoga the Iyengar Way
Silva, Mira & Shyam Mehta . . . .*Simon Schuster 1990*

The Complete Yoga Book
James Hewitt . . . .*Random 1992*

First Steps to Meditation
Lynn Genders . . . .*Axiom 1999*

First Steps to Yoga
Louise Wiggins . . . .*Axiom 1999*

In Stillness I Heal (CD recording)
Louise Wiggins . . . .*Banyan Tree Books 1998*